Foundations for Practice in Occupational Therapy

This book is dedicated to 'the aunts' Muriel I Tarrant-Cunningham and Angela E Rivett-De-Guingaud, founders and co-principals of the London School of Occupational Therapy, to whose vision, inspiration and professionalism I am indebted.

'Without Vision We Perish' (motto of the London School)

For Churchill Livingstone:

Editorial director: Mary Law
Project manager: Valerie Burgess
Project development editor: Valerie Bain
Project controller: Pat Miller
Design direction: Judith Wright
Copy editor: James Dale
Sales promotion executive: Maria O'Connor

Foundations for Practice in Occupational Therapy

Rosemary Hagedorn DipCOT SROT DipTCDHEd MSc
Practising Occupational Therapist, formerly Course Director in Occupational Therapy,
Crawley College of Technology, Crawley, UK

SECOND EDITION

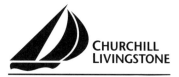

CHURCHILL
LIVINGSTONE

NEW YORK EDINBURGH LONDON MADRID MELBOURNE SAN FRANCISCO TOKYO 1997

CHURCHILL LIVINGSTONE
Medical Division of Pearson Professional Limited

Distributed in the United States of America by Churchill
Livingstone, 650 Avenue of the Americas, New York,
N.Y. 10011, and by associated companies, branches and
representatives throughout the world.

© Pearson Professional Limited 1997

First published 1992
Second edition 1997

ISBN 0 443 0529 2

British Library Cataloguing in Publication Data
A catalogue record for this book is available from the British Library.

Library of Congress Cataloging in Publication Data
A catalog record for this book is available from the Library of Congress.

The
publisher's
policy is to use
**paper manufactured
from sustainable forests**

Printed in the United Kingdom by Bell and Bain Ltd., Glasgow

Contents

Preface

About this book

When I began writing the first edition of this book in 1990, I wanted to provide students and clinical supervisors with a (relatively) simple guide through the murky swamp of 'models and all that'. For many students this was a real 'slough of despond'. Five years later the mud is still sticky, and the bog of ideas just as hard for the novice to move through, although a few points of hard ground are beginning to push above the surface.

Enough of metaphor. I am delighted that the book has proved useful enough to justify a second edition. The original format is retained, but I have tried to update and extend the content in the light of recent developments in theory-building.

If you open this book looking for straightforward 'right or wrong' answers you are still likely to be disappointed. The evolving knowledge base is too complex and contradictory. Our profession remains unable to reach agreement on key definitions and concepts. Perhaps the search for an internationally accepted language for occupational therapy, or a consensus view of an 'OT Paradigm' are simply mirages which distract us from the real business of treating patients? You must decide for yourself.

If you have studied the first edition of *Foundations for Practice* you may be dismayed to find that I have altered some of my ideas and changed my presentation of some concepts. This is partly in response to comments about the original text, and partly because we are all chasing a moving target. This is healthy and adaptive. An individual or profession which fails to change when change is needed is doomed.

About myself

I wish, in this book, to speak directly to you, the reader, in the hope that you will be challenged to think about what you read, to learn actively and not to take all my ideas at face value just because they happen to be in print.

Every author has a past. That past colours and filters perceptions, and produces a personal world complete with beliefs, ideas, blinkers, values and prejudices from which the author cannot escape, even if she tries. I believe that it is important for you to understand that, and to read this book with a critical and questioning attitude.

To that end, it may be useful for you to know a little about my professional background. I qualified in 1965 and worked mainly with adults or older people who had physical disabilities or injuries. As a District Occupational Therapist, I managed a range of services including those for clients with psychosocial or learning disabilities. In 1986 I made a sideways jump into education as Head of the Crawley Occupational Therapy School, where the stimulation of my own academic interests by staff and students led to the writing of this book. Since leaving Crawley, I have continued to write and have taken some time out for personal development (through an MSc in Advanced Occupational Therapy). I have now returned to a mixture of clinical work and research.

I am increasingly convinced that occupational therapy should be overtly based on human occupations, and that the most important core skills of the therapist are occupational analysis and adaptation.

In the preface to the first edition I wrote, 'As a profession we do not spend nearly enough time talking among ourselves about what we actually do and what we really think ... at a time when we are more than ever under the microscope and obliged to justify our services this dialogue is an essential tool in defining our methods, objectives and standards.' This is still true, and I hope that this book will stimulate that discussion.

Arundel 1996   Rosemary Hagedorn

Occupational therapy: an outline of theory and practice

SECTION CONTENTS

1

Introduction

There are now many frames of reference and models to guide the practice of occupational therapy (OT). Getting to grips with the concepts and terminology can be bewildering. What is the use of a model? Is there a difference between a model and a frame of reference? Which one is appropriate in which circumstance? How does theory relate to what the therapist actually does with the patient or client?

The book is intended to form a basic text for students and should also be useful for practising therapists who want to extend their theoretical vocabulary and to take a more analytical approach to their work. It is a book about ideas— the 'whys' and 'whats' of occupational therapy— not about the 'hows' of techniques and practice; for the latter you will need to refer to some of the other sources which I have listed in the references.

The material is presented at introductory level and it is advisable to do additional reading if you intend to put a model into practice. Each section has a list of suggested reading and there is a Bibliography at the end of the book which includes all the references used in the text.

Student therapists often seek guidance on how to treat patients, hoping to be told what is 'right' or 'wrong'. As you gain experience, you realize that planning treatment is seldom that simple. Whilst there may be things which are clearly inappropriate, there are often several possible treatment options. What you select will depend on the individual circumstances and preferences of your patient as much as on the selected model or theory. The skill with which you are able to make this selection depends on the quality of your clinical reasoning; it is not enough to be able to act like a therapist, you also need to learn to think like a therapist.

Examples of potential applications are given in the description of each approach but these should be taken only as indications of possibilities, not as 'formulae'.

If you can relate case studies within your current experience to a particular model or frame of reference, this will help you to understand the application. It can be helpful to imagine what might happen if a different approach were to be used in a particular case. Talk about your ideas with others. There is some discussion in the text and sometimes questions are posed, but do not expect me to give you one 'right' answer: there is almost always more than one, and you may well think of ones which I did not consider.

There is no single 'right' answer

The point about there not being one 'right' answer when we are dealing with frames of reference and models of practice is important. It is comfortable to have the intellectual and emotional assurance of 'being right'. However, the further one progresses with study, the more one discovers that such certainties are few and that even apparently immutable 'facts' may, on close inspection, be subject to doubt. Knowledge continually evolves.

The present state of the art in the area of model building and definition of frames of reference within occupational therapy is still subject to evolution.

You will rapidly discover that ideas are fluid and terms are confusing. Different authors have different versions. This is very challenging to the student, and it also makes it difficult for the person attempting to write a straightforward account of current ideas.

A prominent American educationalist (Perry 1970) has described the developmental process of learning as nine 'Positions', whereby the student makes the difficult cognitive shift from basic dualism (right v. wrong) moving in stages up the scale of conceptualization and the development of meaning, recognizing gradually that it

is legitimate for authorities to hold different opinions. Finally, the student acknowledges that one must develop one's own commitments and yet be flexible enough to change them as learning continues throughout life.

Whether or not you agree with Perry's conceptual model of learning, it may at least be worth remembering that learning produces affective as well as cognitive responses; learning can be stimulating and exciting, but you are also likely to feel confused, challenged or even angry at times as you grapple with new, and sometimes contradictory, concepts.

In Section 1 I describe the use of the occupational therapy process and the core skills of the occupational therapist. I explore the problems of coping with the terminology used in the description of theories and the relationships between theory and practice.

In Section 2 the alternative views of human function and behaviour which form applied frames of reference and their associated approaches are described. Chapter 9 deals with processes of change, and Chapter 10 gives an account of models produced by occupational therapists which provide a view of the individual as a participant in occupations.

This book contains a great deal of condensed information. I hope that it will stimulate your intellectual curiosity and that you will want to read on, but it is probably better to break your reading up into manageable chunks, leaving gaps between 'bites', or you are likely to suffer from the mental equivalent of a bad attack of indigestion!

THE SCOPE OF OCCUPATIONAL THERAPY

Occupational therapy is a complex, broadly based profession, blending medical and social science, merging the artistic and technical aspects of practice.

In part it originates in the eighteenth century with the work of the French physician and psychiatrist Phillipe Pinel and the Englishman William Tuke, who founded The Retreat at York, an asylum in which pioneering and liberal ideas concerning the treatment of the mentally ill were developed.

These ideas, and others, were drawn together around the beginning of the twentieth century in America, where a disparate, and at first scattered, group of professionals — psychiatrists, doctors, nurses, teachers, architects, social workers — evolved the concepts of occupation as a curative agent and of the person as active in promoting his own health and well-being through engagement in occupation. The term 'occupational therapy' was coined by George Barton in 1914 and the National Society for the Promotion of Occupational Therapy (the precursor of the American Association of Occupational Therapy) was founded in 1917.

Definitions abound, and only a few of the more recent ones will be given here.

The World Federation of Occupational Therapists (1989) states that:

Occupational therapy is the treatment of physical and psychiatric conditions through specific activities to help people to reach their maximum level of function and independence.

In 1994 the College of Occupational Therapists (UK) issued a position statement on core skills and the conceptual foundation for practice which gave the WFOT definition and continued:

The occupational therapist assesses the physical, psychological and social functions of the individual, identifies areas of dysfunction and involves the individual in a structured programme of activity to overcome disability. The activities selected will relate to the consumer's personal, social, cultural and economic needs and will reflect the environmental factors which govern his life.

The statement also gives the definition provided by the Committee of Occupational Therapists for the European Community (COTEC):

Occupational therapists assess and treat people using purposeful activity to prevent disability and develop independent function.

Whilst these definitions have the virtue of brevity, they fail to convey the full scope of current OT practice, especially the rapidly developing field of work in the community.

There are many other definitions and explana-

tions, mostly longer, and all subject to criticism. It is an interesting exercise to try to write one's own definition — it gives one a lesson in the problems of constructing a satisfactory, informative summary of something as multifaceted as occupational therapy.

It is, nonetheless, important that therapists are familiar with the available definitions, and essential that each practitioner has a full understanding of the principles, purposes and scope of the profession.

There is still much debate about the nature of occupational therapy, but some consensus concerning the fundamental beliefs and concerns is emerging. Occupational therapy:

- Is concerned with the individual and the roles, occupations, activities and interactions within the individual's personal environment.
- Enables and empowers the individual to be a competent and confident performer in his or her daily life, and enhances his or her well-being.
- Uses activities creatively and therapeutically to achieve goals which are meaningful to the individual and to minimize the effects of dysfunction.
- Requires the individual to engage actively in the process of therapy and to be a partner with the therapist in designing and directing this process.

THE NATURE OF OCCUPATIONAL COMPETENCE AND OCCUPATIONAL DYSFUNCTION

When a person is performing competently he is able to meet the demands of each task, to respond to the demands of each environment, and to use the skills he has learnt in order to act, interact and react appropriately in every situation.

Occupational dysfunction arises when a person is unable to do the normal everyday things which he wants and needs to do. The reasons for this are very variable and may be complex.

A dysfunction is a temporary or chronic inability to engage in the roles, relationships and occupations expected of a person of comparable age, sex and culture. This is not the same as a disability: that tends to imply a loss of physical or cognitive ability, but one may be disabled (e.g. a paraplegic or an amputee) but capable of leading a very functional and adaptive life.

One may be dysfunctional (i.e. maladaptive, unable to cope with the demands of one's life) without having any kind of disability. It is possible for most people to become dysfunctional to some extent when faced with an unfamiliar or difficult situation or when confronted by a very stressful life event, but such dysfunction is usually transient and either resolves when the stress is removed or with minimum intervention. The kind of dysfunction with which occupational therapists deal is often more complex and harder to remedy.

One way of looking at dysfunction is to describe it as a lack of balance between the skills of the individual, the challenges of the environment and the difficulties of the task.

The individual may have lost skills or never learnt them. He may have some negative emotional reaction connected with the activity. The physical environment may be badly designed, too demanding or not demanding enough. The social environment may be too stressful or insufficiently supportive. The task may be too difficult or the tools inappropriate.

The role of the occupational therapist is to intervene to help the individual to balance these factors and regain competence. The therapist can adapt the performance demand of the task, alter the environment to be more supportive, and teach the individual a new repertoire of skills or help him to regain ones he has lost.

Occupational therapy is essentially a process in which the individual must participate actively. The therapist is concerned to enable, empower and enhance, but cannot impose solutions. This

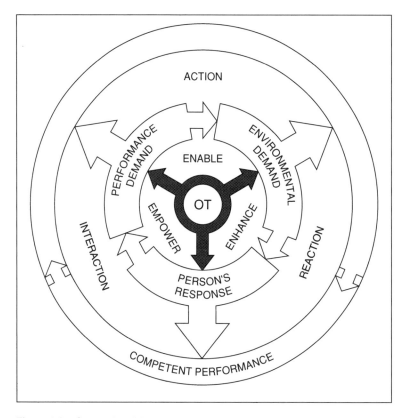

Figure 1.1 Occupational therapy and occupational competence.

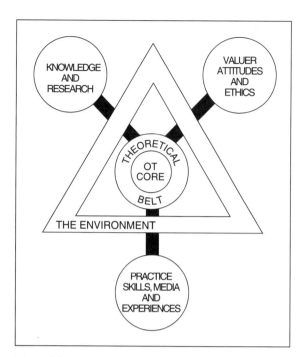

Figure 1.2 Relationships between the elements of professional practice.

The central concept of occupational therapy must, however, somehow be protected and preserved or OT would be in continual danger of either being absorbed by some other profession or changing out of all recognition. This stable, central core has been given many names, as you will see in Chapter 4, including 'paradigm' and 'professional model'.

Around this core are clustered theories and models for practice drawn from many sources. The material in this 'theoretical belt' is influenced both by the content of the core which defines what occupational therapy is, and what it does (and does not do), by the knowledge and research base of the profession, by practitioners' values, attitudes and ethics, and by practice skills, media and experiences.

When a therapist comes to put this into practice what she actually does is further influenced by the environment of practice, which includes the society and culture in which practice takes place, the needs of a particular client group, the location (i.e. in a hospital or in the community), and a host of other contextual factors, including the personal experience of the therapist. This relationship between the elements of professional practice is shown in Figure 1.2.

Perhaps the most challenging concept for students to master is the relationship between the central, stable core of professional practice and the theories which can be used to enable them to understand their patients and to shape their practice in differing situations.

The first section of this book is aimed at exploring and clarifying this important relationship between knowing, doing and thinking.

view of occupational therapy and occupational competence is shown in Figure 1.1.

HOW THEORY RELATES TO PRACTICE

A profession such as occupational therapy must continually develop and evolve in response to the needs of people within a particular culture and in line with developments in science and medicine.

2

The occupational therapy process

The *occupational therapy process* is the name given to the sequence of actions which a therapist undertakes in order to treat a patient. It is not a theory, nor is it therapy, but it provides an organizational structure for both.

There are several representations of this process in the textbooks, each differing a little in accordance with the author's personal concept of the sequence. In general, there is close agreement on the basic format which involves gathering information concerning the patient, her situation and her problems, evaluating this information, defining the aims of therapy, setting priorities for action, deciding on the required action, implementing this and evaluating the outcome.

Although this is commonly called 'the OT process', it is clear that it is not unique to occupational therapy. It is a form of the basic problem solving process which is used by all health care professions.

For example, 'the nursing process', which has been in use for many years, consists of four stages: assessing, planning, implementing and evaluating (Yura & Walsh 1988). The OT process might equally well be described as the process of case management, whereby intervention is defined, sequenced and organized.

As shown in Figure 2.1, a referral is received and this starts the intervention sequence. The therapist will then enter the cycle of information gathering and problem analysis, decision making, implementation of action and review of outcome which is repeated until intervention is judged to be complete and/or the patient is discharged.

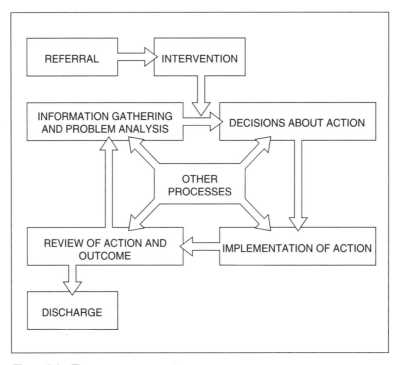

Figure 2.1   The case management process.

So, if this is a generic process used by other professions, what makes it into occupational therapy and not, for example, nursing? The answer is at once simple and very complex; it is an occupational therapist who is using the process. The therapist employs the unique combination of personal experience, knowledge, skills and values which combine to form the practice of occupational therapy. He is able to use the 'OT process' as directed by his clinical reasoning to coordinate and combine other processes. These will be described later, but first the OT process itself requires closer examination.

Representations of the OT process are often either circular or in the form of flow charts, with one stage following neatly from the last. In practice the use of the OT process is more flexible and dynamic than such diagrams suggest.

For one thing, there are subroutines at each stage where information is evaluated, and there are 'escape routes' where it may be decided that intervention is unnecessary or ineffective and should be stopped. Figure 2.2 attempts to depict this more complex, organic form of the problem based OT process.

The student or novice therapist is likely to depend on this sequence quite heavily and must follow it carefully as an aid to clinical reasoning. Studies of expert therapists, however, indicate that with experience the sequence of the OT process becomes 'unhitched' and the therapist is able to move backwards and forwards around the stages in the process as clinical decisions are made, manipulating information in a mental 'problem space' in a manner which requires sophisticated use of clinical reasoning (Mattingly & Fleming 1994; Hagedorn 1995b).

This flexiblity greatly speeds the decision making process, but it requires a cognitive shift which can only be acquired with experience. Students and newly qualified therapists need to spend time mastering the process and consciously using it to structure the delivery of therapy; 'unhitching' is a natural cognitive development which will occur in due course as espertise is acquired, and this development cannot be hurried.

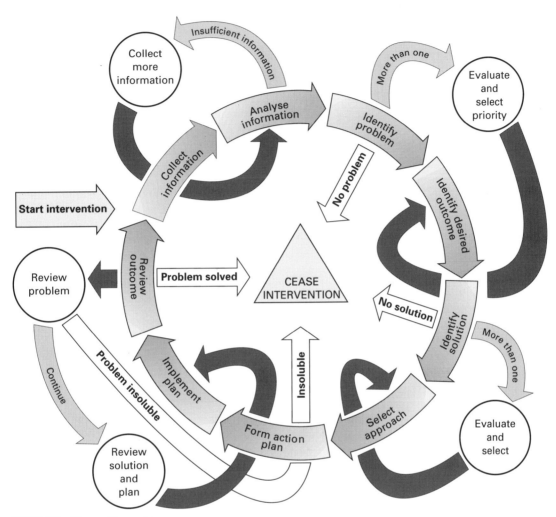

Figure 2.2 The problem solving process.

PROBLEM NAMING, PROBLEM FRAMING AND PROBLEM SOLVING

Problems solving is a basic human skill, and one which is important in therapy. The therapist must discover the nature of the patient's problem and the means of 'solving' it. It is tempting to focus on the element of 'solution'—indeed you will find many references in the literature to 'problem solving'—but it is not possible to solve a problem unless its nature and, perhaps, causation are understood and until you know what outcome your patient would like to achieve.

Naming the problem means 'saying what it is'.

The therapist needs to help his patient to define what is unsatisfactory in the current situation and what, ideally, the patient would like the situation to be.

Framing the problem means choosing to put an interpretation on how to describe and deal with it. For example, 'not going out of the house' could be seen as a problem of mobility, but it might equally be a problem of access (steps in the way), motivation (doesn't want to go out), social isolation (no one to visit) or the result of a specific diagnosis such as agoraphobia. Each interpretation would lead the therapist to take a different course of action to resolve the problem. In some cases more than one frame is applicable, but care must be taken to see that solutions remain compatible.

Once naming and framing have been completed — at least in preliminary form — the therapist and patient can jointly agree on priorities and goals. Only then can the therapist design the means of achieving the desired outcome. The therapist may be equipped with a mental store of 'solutions', but he can only provide an appropriate solution in the context of an individual and her needs.

The problem may turn out to be one familiar to the therapist, or it may be something novel, in which case the therapist must think out a new solution on the basis of his knowledge and experience, or enable the patient to do this for herself — true 'problem solving'.

It may be apparent to the therapist that there is a problem, but the patient may not wish to recognize or deal with this. In fact, getting the patient to accept that there is a problem can *be* the problem.

Conversely, the patient may be experienced by others as having or causing problems whilst the therapist may be able to see that the problem does not lie with the patient, but rather with her physical or social environment, or the nature of the problem task.

It is possible to identify that, although a problem may exist, intervention is unnecessary, ineffective or not beneficial. Some problems are incapable of solution, and many require some compromise or adaptation to be made.

Complex problems may require analysis from a variety of prespectives and theoretical frameworks, each of which may provide a different explanation or course of action. Unravelling such complex situations is very challenging. The skill of finding alternative ways of 'naming and framing' problems is closely linked to the use of models and frames of reference, as will be described later.

COGNITIVE ASPECTS OF PROBLEM SOLVING

Problem solving can be conceptualized as taking place in a mental problem space, a 'box' into which all the available information is put and in which the problem solver manipulates the elements of the problem. 'It contains states of knowledge about the problem. Both the initial situation and the desired situation are represented as elements of this space ... problem solving is always a matter of search' (Newell in Johnson-Laird and Wason 1977).

The problem solver must identify the problem and then find a means of moving from the initial state to a state where the goal is satisfied by means of an operator — some appropriate strategy or action. A heuristic — 'a strategy that can be applied to a variety of problems that usually, but not always, yields a correct solution' (Atkinson 1993) — may be used as an operator. Sometimes problems may be solved by insight, in which the solution is suddenly presented without intervening stages of development.

The problem solver may use means end analysis — a problem solving strategy in which one's current state to the goal state in order to find the most important difference between them. Eliminating this difference then becomes the main subgoal. Another strategy is difference reduction, in which subgoals are set up and achieved, thus moving each time into a state closer to the desired goal (Atkinson 1993).

A familiar solution may become a mental set which may limit problem solving if the problem solver becomes hooked into one particular solution which worked before and cannot change this set when faced with a different, but superficially similar, problem. A patient can become caught in this trap and become unable to see a way out of her difficulty for herself. A therapist must also beware of becoming dependent on familiar solutions to the exclusion of others.

When the problem is complex or unfamiliar, the mind generates a series of 'what if' hypotheses and previously learnt 'rules' which seem applicable and tests these against the desired state. At this stage production of many possible strategies is useful. Good problem solvers are very flexible, have well-developed lateral (divergent) thinking and use strategies such as 'brainstorming' to produce a multitude of creative and novel solutions.

Evaluation and selection of solutions is another key stage in the process: effectiveness may not be the only criterion, for example, one may need to consider acceptability to the client or other's, time, resources, effort, cost and practicality.

The stages in the OT process will now be described in more detail.

Collecting information

The key to problem solution is gathering sufficient information about the situation. This may occupy much of the time spent on the problem and will involve reference to many sources—the patient, other people or professionals, casenotes, textbooks and so forth. Once it is possible to identify accurately what the problem is, a solution is frequently obvious. Attempting to solve a problem which is inadequately understood or where too many assumptions have been made is seldom successful.

Having too much data is often a bigger difficulty than having too little—the ability to select the relevant from the irrelevant comes with experience. Expert judgement and knowledge may be required: the creation of 'expert systems'—computer data bases and diagnostic programmes aimed at helping with clinical problem solving—is a recent development to assist doctors and other professionals. So far there have been few attempts to create expert systems for use by therapists (Arnold & Penn 1990). Information processing is now an important separate branch of knowledge, both in computers and in cognitive psychology.

Problem identification

If the therapist has seen a similar problem before, he can rapidly identify it. Cues are recognized and matched to memories of previous patients and there is a rapid shift from understanding the problem to deciding what could be done about it (this cognitive processing is described in more detail in Ch. 5).

Some situations are unfamiliar or more complex and need more analysis. This involves providing answers to questions such as: what is the problem? Is there more than one? Which is the most significant? Which should be tackled first? The apparent or obvious problem may be a symptom rather than the real cause of the difficulty. Action may turn out to be inadvisable or impossible.

Some people are uncomfortable with the word 'problem': In this context it simply means defining the needs of the patient which are to be the areas for intervention by the occupational therapist (diagnostic reasoning). Putting it another way, the 'problem' is the therapist's initial lack of understanding of the individual and her situation; until sufficient data is gathered, and goals set, action cannot be taken by either the therapist or the patient.

The logical sequence in which problems are tackled is also important—effort can be wasted by dealing with subsidiary issues which would be resolved by solution of the root cause while, on the other hand, the patient may not be ready to tackle 'the big one' but may be able to gain confidence by succeeding with something smaller. Whittling away the peripheral problems with easy solutions can also help to build confidence in the problem solving process and will help to reduce the big problem to a more manageable size. An analogy which can be useful when explaining this to patients is to liken the problem situation to a ladder: it may be too high to reach the top, but if the ladder is sawn down one rung at a time the top will eventually be within reach.

Identification of the desired outcome

Identification of the problem—the 'undesired state' — must bring with it a clear specification of the 'desired state'. This is not the same as a solution, which is the method whereby that state may be achieved and which may sometimes be far more difficult to identify. The desired outcome may be clear, but the route to it hard to find.

Much depends on the patient's perceptions of her needs. Defining the desired outcome requires negotiation between therapist and patient. Goals should never be imposed.

Often there is only one desired outcome, but sometimes there may be alternatives, which can be evaluated for comparative benefits, put in priority order, discarded or kept in reserve as a viable alternative if the first choice proves unattainable.

Goal setting is an essential prerequisite for therapy or intervention, and it is often necessary to define goals in terms of timescale — immediate or longer term, and to subdivide them into objectives. An objective should contain a clear statement of what is to be achieved and some means of measuring the outcome.

Problem identification and decisions about the desired outcome involve diagnostic reasoning, which is described in the section on clinical reasoning.

Solution development, evaluation and selection

The human brain is uniquely geared to be effective at problem solving. At a low level it can do this so rapidly that it appears intuitive, although this is actually based on fast processing of previous knowledge and experience together with insightful connective 'jumps' between pieces of information.

The more experienced the therapist, the bigger his mental stock of available solutions and actions will be. Students, however, lack this resource and will inevitably take longer to sort out what to do.

Again, possible actions need to be checked out with the patient, and her approval must be gained. Actions which a patient clearly rejects, however beneficial, cannot be carried out.

Development of an action plan

The *action plan* specifies the stages by which the solution will be implemented and the desired state achieved. It should also make it clear who is responsible for doing what. Although the plan should not become too rigid, clarity in specifying the goal, timescale and method of testing success or failure is helpful and assists outcome measurement.

An action plan may relate to action by the therapist, but it may equally well define action to be taken by the patient or others.

Implementation

The plan is put into action and the process and results are recorded. It is important to keep checking that the plan is moving towards the target. The therapist must keep in mind any service standards or quality statements to ensure that practice meets these requirements. All interventions must be well documented.

Evaluation of results

The effectiveness of the action is measured against progress towards the previously agreed outcome. Once that is achieved, intervention ceases or moves to another problem. Compromises may be necessary. Action may uncover previously unsuspected problems which need to be dealt with. Action which is ineffective must be changed. Was the solution wrong? Was the problem incorrectly defined in the first place? Is the problem insoluble, or the gain not worth prolonged effort? Answers to these questions usually require a return circuit round the problem solving process, gathering more information and redefining the problem.

PROBLEM BASED RECORDING SYSTEMS

'Problem solving' is often associated with problem based systems of recording, particularly problem oriented medical records (POMR) (Weed 1968; 1969) and the SOAP system.

Problem oriented medical records

Using this system, the problems experienced by the patient are identified and listed. They may be categorized under headings according to a standardized system and may be allocated numbers. Once listed, problems are prioritized and may be divided into short-term and long-term goals. A treatment plan is designed and implemented for selected goals. It is useful to separate the **treatment plan** which will involve the patient's direct participation from the **action plan**, which is what the therapist (or others) will do. All references to the treatment and subsequent progress in resolving the problem refer to it by number. When the problem is resolved, it is removed from the list and subsequent problems may be tackled (Kings Fund Centre 1988).

Putting this recording system into practice requires some effort, but once set up it does aid teamwork and concentrates efforts on practical issues by identifying the action to be taken and the most appropriate person to take it, and facilitating review of progress.

SOAP

SOAP is a method of problem identification and solution, SOAP stands for:

Subjective
Objective
Assessment (or Analysis)
Planning

First, the patient's subjective view of her situation is obtained and recorded, together with the subjective views of any other people involved.

Following this, the therapist will identify some likely problem areas and investigate these objectively by formal observation and assessments.

The results of these procedures will then be analysed in order to decide what the problem(s) might be. At this stage it may become clear that the patient's subjective view differs from the objective assessment of the therapist or from the subjective views of significant others and this mismatch may in fact constitute the problem. Once a problem list has been composed it is possible to decide on action.

The planning stage involves selecting priorities, goal setting, generating possible solutions and selecting the preferred one, and putting the plan into action, as described earlier in this chapter.

Although SOAP does not contain another stage, it is implicit that the success of the plan is monitored and reviewed and action modified accordingly. The number of 'problems solved' at the end of the intervention can be used as an outcome measure.

When using this system, all actions by the therapist are recorded with the key letters S,O,A,P. For example, an interview with the patient would be under S; an observation of the occurrence of a particular difficulty would be under O, together with the number of the problem observed; a case conference might be A or P; the treatment plan would be P.

Using this system does take practice and requires a certain mental discipline, but once proficiency is attained it can greatly speed up and simplify the process of keeping treatment records, as well as making goal setting and planning more precise. It also offers the advantage of a measurable outcome which is of considerable value in implementing quality assurance audits and producing evidence of the results of therapy.

There can be difficulties in fitting actions or occurrences into the SOAP format, and the system should not be allowed to get in the way of good recording. Some forms of problem based systems include a 'strengths and needs' assessment of the individual — Individual Programme Planning is an example — so that strengths can be built on as part of the problem solving process. This also avoids the risk of a rather negative 'problem list' which may result in the patient being viewed as 'a problem'.

POMR and SOAP may be linked to a 'key worker' system, where an individual is given the responsibility of managing a case and coordinating effective therapy.

3

Core skills and processes

Occupational therapists use different approaches and techniques depending on the speciality and location in which each therapist works, and their experience. There may appear to be little in common between the therapist who assesses the home for the provision of an adapted ground floor extension, the one who takes a session of psychodrama and the one who rehabilitates a patient's hand function following a severe crush injury.

What, then, is occupational therapy and how does its practice differ from that of similar professions? Is practice purely contextual and a matter of individual style? Good multidisciplinary teamwork frequently encourages blurring of professional boundaries—it matters less who does it than that it is done effectively. But if it does not matter, and if anyone can do the job, who needs the therapist?

'What do we do that is different?' is a central question for any profession. If the question is not answered for occupational therapy it becomes difficult to define the body of knowledge or the standard of skill which students must acquire if they are to become competent practitioners. It is also difficult to define and defend service provision, to set and maintain standards, to ensure quality or to ensure that occupational therapists' skills are used to best effect, which is of increasing importance when therapists are in short supply.

For these reasons there has been considerable interest, both from the profession and its managers, in identifying and describing core skills and 'skill mix'. This process is not without its dangers. If carried to extremes, it can become reductive and therapy may come to be regarded as a mechanistic process more at a technician's level than that of a professional practitioner.

As discussed in the keynote address at the World Federation of Occupational Therapists' Congress (Barnitt 1990): The attempt to define the knowledge, skills and attitudes which form the structure of the profession may lead us towards adopting standardized practices and formulae which actually inhibit thinking and dynamic professional development. Our core skills must, somehow, encompass the nebulous aspects of professional judgement, problem solving and research as well as the 'hands on' forms of therapeutic knowledge and skill.

Work on clinical reasoning which has taken place since that Congress has greatly added to our understanding of the alchemy which transmutes a selection of generic and special skills into occupational therapy.

A core skill may be defined as one of the essential elements of professional practice the use of which remains relatively constant, although adapted by the selection of therapeutic models or frames of reference.

> **Q** Before going any further, write down your own list of occupational therapy core skills — the things which are essential for effective practice. When you have your list, next divide the skills listed into those which *only* occupational therapists use, or use in a unique way, and those which other medical or paramedical professions use. If you can, compare your list with someone else's — do they differ? How, and why?

WHAT ARE OCCUPATIONAL THERAPISTS' CORE SKILLS?

There is still a debate within the profession over what constitutes legitimate and 'illigitimate' professional practice, but a consensus is beginning to develop.

It has to be remembered that all such analysis is artificial; in practice therapy operates as a total package, a gestalt. Most attempts at defining the skills required to practice occupational therapy are made, consciously or unwittingly, from the perspective of the writer's speciality and preferred structure, which will bring with them specific skills and emphasize specific aspects. Such definitions often fail to distinguish between those elements which are generic and those which are derived from the particular structure and circumstances.

Mosey, for example, states that:

a profession is characterized by a description of six elements: the profession's philosophical assumptions, ethical code, body of knowledge, domain of concern, nature of and principles for sequencing the various aspects of practice, and the profession's legitimate tools.

She gives an account of these 'tools' in the context of psychosocial occupational therapy (Mosey 1986).

In the first edition of this book (1992), I produced a list of core skills, subdivided into:

● **Generic core skills.** Those skills which are common to the treatment process employed by occupational therapists and other similar health care professions. Occupational therapists will put their own professional slant on these skills, but they are not radically changed when used by different professions, and at the level of basic training much of the knowledge base could be shared.
● **Primary core skills.** Those managerial, interactive and therapeutic skills which are specific to occupational therapy or which occupational therapists use in a way which is particular to the profession.

I used the word *skill* as a convenient shorthand to mean 'a learnt ability and applied knowledge used to achieve a task to a definable standard of competence'.

I subdivided core skills into three groups in each section:

● managerial skills
● interactive skills
● therapeutic skills.

Whilst this seemed a useful arrangement at the time, it was somewhat complex and there was some difficulty in allocating core skills to each of these categories. In the light of subsequent developments which have provided more consensus concerning the nature of core skills (as shown by Table 3.1), it seems preferable to abandon this three part classification, although the distinction between generic and unique skills is worth exploring.

In a subsequent publication (Hagedorn 1995b) I have described in more detail a list of seven core processes—more complex, integrated forms of skill—under the headings of :

- case management (including problem solving and clinical reasoning)
- assessment and evaluation
- therapeutic use of self
- analysis and adaptation of occupations
- analysis and adaptation of environments
- intervention (provision of therapy or other action)
- resource management.

For me the truly unique processes are environmental and occupational analysis and adaptation; the College of Occupational Therapists' list of skills (1994) also accepts this view. I believe that the other skills and processes are to a greater or lesser extent generic in that they are used in similar form by other professions. What is

unique is the combination of these processes as applied by an occupational therapist in an individual case.

I will therefore describe generic skills in general terms, and then primary core skills and processes in more detail.

GENERIC CORE SKILLS

Organizational skills, e.g. independent management of self and own resources; routine administration, appointments systems; planning delivery of services; delegating work to assistants; monitoring workload.

Financial skills, e.g. effective, efficient and economical provision of services; budget monitoring; ordering; stocktaking.

Recording skills, e.g. selecting relevant information; clear concise record-keeping which is comprehensible to others; using correct language and format; recording at appropriate intervals; keeping statistical records; maintaining confidentiality.

Research skills, e.g. able to undertake literature searches; understand basic research methodology, both quantitative and qualitative; formulate proposals for research projects; undertake interviews; construct questionnaires; under-

Table 3.1 Comparison of lists of core skills

Mosey (1986) (legitimate tools)	Reed (1992) (service provisions)	Willard and Spackman (1992) (tools of practice)	COT (1994) (skills)
Use of the non-human environment	Use of normal or adapted environments	Environmental adaptation	Assess and manipulate environments
Conscious use of self		Therapeutic use of self	
The teaching-learning process	Teaching		
Use of purposeful activities	Use of normal activities	Use of activity and activity analysis	Therapeutic use of purposeful activity
Use of activity groups	Use of activity groups	Group process	
Activity analysis and synthesis	Use of adapted activities and task analysis	(Activity analysis)	Analysis and application of activities
Assessment and evaluation	Assessment and evaluation Use of adaptive equipment	Assessment and evaluation Assisted and adaptive equipment: use of technology Service management Research	

stand and use simple statistics; produce material for professional journals.

Problem solving skills, use of basic problem solving methodology, e.g. strategies to define and analyse problem; select priorities for action; produce and correctly evaluate possible solutions; select optimum solution; plan and carry out action; evaluate results; redefine problem and plan new action if required.

Communication skills, e.g. verbal skills; telephone skills; use of information technology; written communications; formal and informal communication methods — at professional level; with patients, carers and lay people, group and dyadic.

Supervisory skills, supervise assistants and students; coordinate the work of others.

Teaching skills, e.g. prepare and use visual aids; construct training programmes; give lectures; demonstrate and instruct students.

Basic counselling skills, e.g. non-verbal skills; listening; reflecting; cueing; prompting.

Basic group skills, awareness of group process; aware of a range of purposes and types of groups; able to organize, run and monitor therapeutic groups; use of appropriate leadership styles; able to act as co-therapist.

Patient care skills, e.g. preservation of individual rights and dignity; awareness of individual needs; safe handling and lifting; correct choice and use of mobility aids; patient comfort and correct positioning; basic personal care, e.g. assistance with eating or use of toilet; maintenance of safe procedures and environment.

Observation skills, take account of physical appearance of patient; facial expression, posture, dress; observe external changes of medical significance, e.g. skin colour, sweating, condition of scar; observe interactions, e.g. patterns or frequency of communication, non-verbal signals; consistent relationships; note environmental content; notice hazards.

PRIMARY CORE SKILLS AND PROCESSES

Case management

Planning therapy or intervention is a managerial

task in two senses: firstly, in 'managing' the patient or client's condition, needs or problem; and secondly, in effectively coordinating all the aspects of the therapist's personal knowledge and resources with those of others.

The ability to make correct decisions about what to do, to decide on priorities, set aims and objectives, plan how these are to be achieved, and to implement these decisions efficiently (i.e. to employ the OT process) requires the development and use of clinical reasoning in a manner which is unique to occupational therapists. Although the process is one used by others (as already noted), the synthesis of knowledge and skill through reasoning results in occupational therapy.

The case management process is influenced by the selection of a model or applied frame of reference. It includes setting standards, monitoring practice, and evaluating outcomes.

Setting standards and evaluating outcomes

The maintenance of personal and professional standards is a prime responsibility of any practitioner and can only be judged in relation to the profession's specific knowledge base and primary core skills. Therapy must be evaluated to ensure that it is effective and to justify continuing or discontinuing therapy/intervention. The therapist should set standards, communicate treatment results to others, be critical of their own performance, monitor and audit quality of service, seek regular supervision, evaluate and update personal knowledge.

OT managers have become concerned to find a means of measuring outcomes in order to judge the efficacy of therapy. This is more difficult than it sounds and there is still much debate about how it can be done.

It is also important to have some means of measuring competence against a defined criterion. Some professional associations have published lists of standards and competencies; those of the American Association are especially well defined (see Hopkins & Smith [Willard and Spackman Occupational Therapy] 1993).

Therapeutic use of self

In nursing, social work or the remedial professions, the dyadic therapeutic relationship between the professional and the patient/client is of great importance. The basic skills of listening, observing non-verbal cues and adapting responses are required by all health care practitioners.

Whilst occupational therapists frequently engage in ordinary dyadic interactions, the process of occupational therapy is unique in that the relationship may be considered not as a dyad (therapist/patient) but as a *triad* (therapist/patient/occupation). The occupation/activity is the medium whereby the interaction is enabled or explored.

Whether working with an individual or with a group, the therapist's awareness of personal attributes and skills in interpersonal relationships and the sensitive and empathetic use of such attributes or skills in the context of an activity or task in order to develop a therapeutic relationship with the participant(s), and to achieve a therapeutic goal, is at the centre of the practice of occupational therapy.

The use of this process could include the following skills:

- Select and enhance features of an activity to promote specific interactions.
- Decide on degree of direction/non-direction/leadership style.
- Use knowledge of group process appropriately.
- Allow or restrict personal spontaneity.
- Control use of humour.
- Set limits for self.
- Be aware of own emotions and reactions: consciously use these for positive therapeutic purposes or avoid negative effects on therapy.
- Understand own attitudes and prejudices and possible effects on relationships; avoid being judgemental.
- Define and adhere to own meaning of 'professional behaviour' and 'ethics'.
- Monitor self and be aware of own needs.
- Be aware of dangers of manipulating or dominating others.
- Give patient appropriate reactions, e.g. praise, encouragement, consolation.

- Use confidence in self to give patient confidence and trust in treatment.
- Use personal initiative, imagination, creativity.

Assessment skills

Assessment of levels of performance in occupational areas, and of occupational roles and skills comprises a large part of OT practice. The type of assessment used and the objectives of the assessment will relate to the needs of the patient and the approach within which the therapist is operating (see Appendix 1 for a list of assessments related to different approaches). Students should note that in American texts the words *evaluation* and *assessment* mean the opposite to the meanings generally given in English text—yet another source of confusion!

It is acknowledged that the basic skills of assessment (e.g. select what is to be assessed; select or design correct assessment methods; be objective; show good observation skills; produce consistent, accurate and, where possible, replicable, results; communicate results clearly to others; be sensitive to the patient as an individual not an object) are used by other professions, but in the context of OT, a crucial primary core skill is the ability to conduct assessments and to analyse the results in order to plan therapy or intervention in an area of occupational performance or dysfunction. Assessments may be conducted within an applied frame of reference or model, or as a means of selecting one.

Assessment should be recognized as a means to an end—identification of the problem; definition of a starting point for treatment/intervention; measurement of progress; evaluation of outcome—not as an end in itself. There is little value in defining a problem if it is not then possible to offer to do something about it.

Assessment may be formal or informal, be used once, or sequentially, and can utilise a wide variety of techniques. Assessment involves:

- information gathering
- observation
- measurement

- recording
- evaluation against a norm or outcome.

Assessment methodology

There is extensive literature about the structure and methods of assessment. Assessments need to be valid and reliable.

Validity concerns whether the assessment actually deals with matters which are appropriate to the situation and measures the right things.

Face validity means that it looks as if the assessment does these things, but it has not been proved to do so. Scientific validity has to be tested and proved by formal research involving control groups, using researched and accepted norms of performance, and tested for statistical validity.

Reliability means that you can be sure that, provided the assessment is used correctly, each time the test is used (test–retest reliability) and whoever uses it (inter-rater reliability), the results can be depended upon. Gaining evidence of reliability in scientific terms is another difficult and time-consuming process involving much research.

Formats for assessment

Assessments may be:

Standardized. Usually conducted following a format which has been piloted on a reasonably large sample of subjects and adjusted for inter-rater reliablity. There is an explicit standard against which the results of the assessment can be judged. There are numerous standardized and validated tests on the market, particularly in the areas of cognition, intelligence, perception, personality and performance skills. Some of these would be of use to occupational therapists but can only be purchased following special training.

Informal. Ad hoc, unstandardized tests; assessments based on subjective observation in normal environments. Many assessments are constructed by occupational therapists and whilst these employ questionnaires, checklists, grading systems and structured performance tests few are standardized and very few properly validated — not least because this requires detailed research, large samples of patients and control groups, and because it is an extremely complex and time-consuming procedure which is beyond the scope of most busy practitioners.

Single or sequential. An assessment may be a 'one off' exercise, or a sequential process where the same performance is reassessed at intervals. In either case there may be a standardized measure, or the individual's previous performance or 'normal' performance where this is observable can be used as the base line.

Objective or subjective. It is impossible (outside of laboratory conditions, and perhaps even then) to be totally objective. Some performances can be assessed with reasonable consistency against known criteria, but many cannot. The criteria do not exist; the effects of environment, the therapist/patient relationship, the mood and motivation of the patient, the skills, expectations, attitudes and intentions of the observer and the well documented effects of the process of being observed on the performance of the subject, all have the potential to alter, or at worst invalidate, assessment results. In the context of OT, it may have to be accepted that intuitive methods of assessment, based on experience and professional judgement, can be valid.

The patient's understanding of his problem is often revealing, and some assessments are designed to elicit this subjective view.

Assessment procedures

All assessment procedures require a basis of theoretical knowledge and practical experience and expertise. Basic methods may be used in a variety of ways, formal and informal. The subject may be asked to perform an action or complete a task, or to complete a self-rating form. Alternatively, the therapist investigates or measures, whilst the subject is relatively passive.

Procedures for obtaining information:

- *Interviews*: informal and unstructured or formal and structured.
- *Questionnaires*: self-rating or administered.

- *Performance tests*: physical; cognitive; interactive. The subject completes a task or demonstrates skill or knowledge.
- *Measurement techniques*: frequently of physical function.
- *Observation and sampling techniques*: to obtain a profile of the subject.

Procedures for collating and evaluating information:

- *Rating scales*: giving a grading or numerical score.
- *Checklists*: as a structured aid to observation.
- *Record forms*: a structured aid to observation and sequential comparison.
- *Charts, grids or graphs*: a visual aid to recording and evaluating results.
- *Statistical formulae*: to evaluate significance of data.
- *Profiling*: provides a comprehensive 'picture'of the subject.

Intervention

Therapy means treatment, which is something which involves the patient and normally requires his active participation. It follows that much of the action is taken by the patient, although it may be initiated or facilitated by the therapist.

Direct treatment is not always required, and frequently there is the need for some action by the therapist which does not involve participation by the patient, hence the use of the term 'intervention'. Studies have shown that between 50% and 30% of a therapist's time may be spent in actions which are not direct 'hands on/face to face' patient treatment.

For example, the therapist may need to conduct interviews, write letters or make contact with a wide range of agencies which may assist the patient, obtain equipment, plan adaptations, communicate with relatives or make visits. In the case of the community based therapist, the latter aspects are likely to form the major part of the therapist's intervention, and may be recorded in the form of an 'action plan' rather than a therapeutic programme.

For simplicity, the word *intervention* will be used in this text to cover therapy and other forms of action.

Intervention may require the therapist to use a repertoire of personal skills.

Therapeutic skills

Technical and creative skills

Occupational therapists require a personal repertoire of practical and creative skills at a sufficient level of competence to provide safe, flexible, imaginative and effective therapy in a range of situations and with different specialities. Skills and techniques may include knowledge of and ability to carry out/teach technical and creative processes and activities used in work, leisure or self-care.

Typical skills include:

- Trade and technical skills, e.g. woodwork, metalwork, horticulture, printing, computer operation, typing, word-processing.
- Craft skills, e.g. weaving, rugmaking, macrame, pottery, sewing.
- Creative and expressive skills, e.g. art, collage, drama, mime, puppetry, music, dance, creative writing.
- Domestic skills, e.g. cooking, budgeting, menu planning, domestic activities, 'Do It Yourself', garden maintenance.
- Leisure skills, sport, hobbies, recreational activities, games, 'keep fit', outings.

Specialist skills and techniques

All therapists require a basic repertoire of specialist skills. Whilst these will develop with experience, basic practitioners typically have some experience in a representative range of techniques.

Examples may include abilities to:

- Make and fit orthoses.
- Instruct in use of prostheses.
- Assess for, provide and train in the use of wheelchairs.
- Adapt or provide therapeutic apparatus and assistive equipment for use in activities of daily living, work or leisure.

- Make recommendations for the provision of housing adaptations for disabled people.
- Use neurodevelopmental handling, positioning and stimulation techniques (e.g. Bobath, PNF, sensorimotor techniques)
- Test and retrain perceptual-motor function.
- Use behavioural modification techniques.
- Conduct social skills training.
- Use reminiscence and reality orientation.
- Use projective techniques and media including music, art, creative writing, bibliotherapy.
- Use psychodrama, role-play, guided fantasy and related techniques.

Some of these techniques will be learnt within the context of specific frames of reference for which they are appropriate. For example, projective techniques may be associated with an analytical frame of reference, whilst Bobath technique would be used within a neurodevelopmental frame of reference.

Therapeutic knowledge

Ability to apply factual and theoretical knowledge

OT requires a synthesis of knowledge, some of which is derived from basic sciences and some is generated by and specific to occupational therapy. Although many of the individual components studied are shared by other professions, the precise emphasis and combination of subjects is unique to OT. Subjects studied normally include: anatomy, physiology, kinesiology, ergonomics, medicine, surgery, psychiatry, psychology, sociology, learning theory, human occupations, theory and practice of occupational therapy.

The assimilation and integration of this knowledge enables a therapist to:

- Comprehend the nature of traumatic or pathological processes affecting the individual.
- Comprehend the nature and causes of dysfunction in occupational performance.
- Make correct professional judgements to determine treatment aims and methods and to predict outcomes.

- Select and analyse treatment techniques, using and adapting activities as required.
- Treat the patient safely and effectively.
- Undertake research.
- Use professional literature constructively and with comprehension.
- Communicate with members of other professions.

ANALYSIS AND ADAPTATION OF OCCUPATIONS

Terminology

In Chapter 4 the problems of using words such as 'model', 'paradigm' or 'frame of reference' will be discussed. It is impossible to describe occupational analysis without coming across another controversial set of definitions: what exactly is meant by 'occupation', 'activity' and 'task'?

One might imagine that these words would by now have been provided with stable, accepted definitions, but unfortunately this is not so. They tend to be used in the texts rather casually, as if they were synonyms.

For example, the word *activity* tends to be used when trying to define occupation:

Any goal directed activity that has meaning for the individual and is composed of skills and values (Creek 1990).

Activities or tasks that engage a person's resources of time and energy. Specifically, self-maintenance, productivity and leisure activities (Reed 1992).

Specific chunks of activity within the ongoing stream of human behaviour which are named in the lexicon of the culture (Yerxa et al).

The latter definition is closer to my own view which is that:

An occupation is a structured form of human endeavour which has a name and associated role title. It provides longitudinal organization of time and effort in a person's life (Hagedorn 1995a).

'Occupation' is a convenient shorthand to use when we want to encompass the whole of human productive endeavour, as in the professional title, but an occupation is too large an entity to be used in therapy; it is lived or experienced, not performed. Indeed, most OT texts speak of activities rather than occupations when they describe therapeutic application, and this has provoked an energetic debate over whether the profession should be named occupational therapy or activity therapy. (Practitioners in the European Community who use the term 'Ergotherapy' are spared this problem, but should not ignore the debate.)

The American OT Association's view of the meaning of the word 'occupation' and associated terminology is set out in a position paper (AJOT (1995) 49 (10): 115–117). They also admit that whilst words associated with occupations 'such as actions, tasks and projects' imply differences in complexity '... there is little agreement among scholars in occupational therapy or the social sciences for how these terms ought to be used to describe various levels of complexity in occupational behaviour'.

I view occupations, activities and tasks as arranged in an hierarchy in which tasks are the basic units of performance and activities are more complex arrangements of tasks. An activity takes place on a specific occasion, during a finite period, for a specific purpose and a completed activity results in a change in the previous state of objective reality or subjective experience. Activities are the means whereby a person is able to experience and change the environment (for definitions refer to the glossary).

It must be said that this is not yet a generally accepted view; many other authorities continue to use the words as synonyms, and a few reverse my definition, viewing tasks as I view activities.

This confusion is regrettable, but, like the confusion over theoretical terminology, it should not be allowed to get in the way of understanding the process of activity analysis. It is, however, important that the student realizes that words may not be used in the same way in different texts. The following description relates to my own definitions, as just described.

Analysis and adaptation of occupations: purposes

The analysis of occupations and their prescription as therapy are the unique skills of the occu-

pational therapist. The analysis and prescription of occupations have two purposes:

- To deal with problems experienced by the patient in all aspects of his or her everyday life, or with social roles (e.g. parent, friend, citizen). These aspects of normal living are usually classified as work, leisure and self-care (ADL).
- The use of activities as specific therapeutic media to treat dysfunctions in the performance of occupations, interactions and roles.

Solving performance problems

The occupational therapist uses a variety of techniques to assess abilities and deficits, to retrain skills and to problem solve in these occupational areas. The individuals requiring this service are frequently those who are disabled rather than dysfunctional. Once environmental constraints are removed or methods of using residual skills to best advantage have been mastered, such individuals can become independent and contributing members of society. Therapists working in the community are likely to spend much of their time in solving performance problems and adapting environments.

Application of activities as therapy

The selection of a therapeutic activity requires that a balance be achieved between the needs and interests of the patient, the personal repertoire of skills possessed by the therapist and the requirements of the model or approach within which the therapist chooses to work. Activities should be specifically selected for the individual patient with a view to a defined goal, e.g.:

- assessing ability
- meeting a need
- solving a problem
- providing experience
- improving a skill
- stimulating an interest
- promoting independence
- encouraging an interaction

- stimulating exploration
- providing opportunities for choice.

Activities may be used casually for recreation, or as pastimes; such use is perfectly valid in the right context. This may be called diversional occupation, *but it is not occupational therapy.*

Whilst engaging the patient in prescribed remedial activities remains a central professional skill, for many therapists it may play a relatively small part in their interventions, which will be concerned more with the analysis of dysfunction in occupational areas and the consequent problem solving actions, as described above.

Techniques of analysis, adaption and application

There are two aims for occupational analysis:

- To understand the nature of an individual's participation and performance and what it means to him. This is focused on the person as 'doer' and enables problems and needs to be understood and treatment goals to be set (performance analysis, participation analysis, existential analysis).
- To understand the nature of the occupation, activity or task. This is focused on the thing to be done and is necessary when selecting or adapting some aspect as therapy or trying to gain a better understanding of what the occupation, activity or task involves (occupational analysis, activity analysis, task analysis, applied analysis).

Participation analysis and existential analysis

Participation analysis (concerned with the range and frequency of participation) and *existential analysis* (concerned with subjective meanings associated with the activity) are techniques which are still developing (Kielhofner 1995; Hagedorn 1995a). They may concern: examination and description of the scope of an individual's existing, past or required occupations; analysing occupations in terms of roles; analysing the socio-cultural importance or meaning of an occupation for the individual.

Performance analysis

This is concerned with the degree to which the person is able to do what he wants and needs to do, is well established, and often focuses on identifying problems in personal and domestic activities of daily living or employment.

Identification of patient problem may include:

- Observing patient performing task in realistic environment and context.
- Defining and recording skills used, level of competence and problem area(s).
- Examining problem in subtask if required.
- Considering social/cultural factors if relevant.
- Considering roles of participant(s).
- Proposing likely cause(s) of dysfunction, e.g. learning difficulty, developmental disorder, skill deficit, lack of practice, role rejection.

Occupational analysis

This may include: contextual evaluation of whether the occupation is work, leisure or self-care. The therapist's traditional division of occupations into work, leisure or activities of daily living must be acknowledged as artificial: in practice the edges blur. Classification is contextual — what one person regards as a chore may be a hobby for someone else. Is housework work or self-care? This method of division, and particularly the currently popular concept that life should contain an appropriate balance of the three occupational areas, is biased towards developed Western-style cultures and may require considerable modification in cultures where such distinctions break down. However, it remains a convenient method of analysis.

Work. Any problem which prevents an individual who wishes to work from doing so is likely to have considerable social, psychological and economic consequences. The therapist may use industrial therapy, work related rehabilitation, adaptation of the workplace and preliminary vocational guidance and training to assist return to work. More complex vocational guidance and retraining is not within the scope of the therapist.

Leisure. Awareness of self-actualization needs

and the importance of the quality of life is increasing, and a proportion of the people who are unemployed and of the growing number of retired people find it hard to cope with unstructured time and need guidance, whilst for those who are unable to work due to a disability or illness, leisure may become crucial in giving purpose and meaning to life.

Activities of daily living (ADL). These activities range from those fundamental for survival (personal activities of daily living (PADL)) — eating, keeping warm, avoiding danger, maintaining personal hygiene and, in some settings, basic social skills — to the more complex aspects of personal self-care and independent living such as cooking, shopping and housework (domestic activities of daily living (DADL) also known in the USA as instrumental activities of daily living (IADL)).

Assessment is carried out to identify the nature and severity of the problem. A programme of practice and training is then provided in as realistic a setting as possible. Any residual disabilities which persist after a period of training are resolved by the provision of adapted equipment, environmental adaptation, or assistance for the individual.

Activity analysis

This involves dissecting the activity into its component parts (tasks) and sequence, looking at its stable and situational components and evaluating its therapeutic potential.

A preliminary analysis will consider the basic content of the activity in terms of, for example:

- The kinds(s) of performance needed to achieve the activity — e.g. cognitive, motor, interpersonal (the headings used for detailed analysis will depend on the approach being used, or a comprehensive analysis may be attempted).
- The degree of complexity of the activity.
- The positive or negative social or cultural associations.
- Whether the activity is structured or unstructured.

- Defining the tasks of which the activity is comprised.
- Analysing the sequence of task performance and whether this is fixed or flexible.
- Defining the tools, furniture, materials and environment required for completion of the activity.
- Defining and taking account of safety precautions or risk factors.

Task analysis

Similarly, this involves a detailed analysis, breaking down the task into subtasks and analysing the general categories of motor, cognitive, perceptual or interactive skills required at each stage or at a particular stage. This may include an analysis of specific movements and the types of muscle action or groups of muscles used to produce these. There are two main purposes for this exercise, either to select an appropriate task to meet a therapeutic aim or objective, or as a means of analysing the precise area of, or cause of, a performance problem.

Skill analysis

Conducting a full analysis of all the skills or subskills required to perform a particular task can be complex and time consuming. A task is performed as a gestalt, and 'unpacking' the components of performance or identifying the relationships between these and causes of dysfunction is not easy. The process is normally conducted by means of close observation and the use of knowledge of anatomy, physiology, perception, cognition, learning theory and theories of human interactions. It is usual to impose some kind of structure on such an analysis. Setting norms for performance is also difficult and is the object of research; unfortunately the 'super fit' population frequently chosen for such studies renders the data inapplicable for most OT purposes. A list of headings used in skill analysis is given in Table 3.2. All these lists contain further subdivisions, which indicates the complexity of skill analysis or assessment. Although authors have

Table 3.2 Examples of taxonomies of performance skills

Model of human occupation (Kielhofner 1995 ch8)	Adaptation through occupation (Reed 1992 pp 124–139)	Adaptive skills (Mosey 1986 p. 42 Table 3.1)
Motor	*Sensorimotor*	*Sensory integration*
Posture	Sensory awareness	Integration of tactile subsystems
Mobility	Sensory processing	Postural and bilateral integration
Coordination	Perceptual	Praxis
Strength and effort	Motor	
Energy	Neuromuscular	
Process	*Cognitive*	*Cognitive function*
Energy	Level of arousal	Attention, memory and orientation
Knowledge	Orientation	Thought processes
Temporal organization	Attending behaviour	Levels of conceptualization
Organizing space and objects	Attention span	Intelligence
Adaptation	Recognition	Factual information
	Memory	Problem solving
	Reality testing	
	Association	
	Categorization	
	Concept formation	
	Sequencing	
	Problem solving	
	Judgement of safety	
	Generalization of learning	
	Integration of learning	
	Synthesis of learning	
	Time management	
Communication and interaction	*Psychosocial*	*Social interaction*
Physicality	Social:	Interpretation of situations
Language		Social skills
Relations	Social conduct	Structured social interplay
Information exchange	Socialization and conversation	
	Role behaviour	
	Dyadic interaction	
	Group interaction	
	Interpersonal relationships	
Social interaction	*Psychological:*	*Psychological function*
Acknowledging	Role identity	Dynamic states
Sending	Self concept	Intrapsychic dynamics
Timing	Locus of control	Reality testing
Coordinating	Mood	Insight
	Initiation/termination of activity	Object relations
	Coping skills	Self-concept
	Self-control	Self-discipline
	Self-efficacy	
	Self-expression	

used different taxonomies, it is possible to see similarities between the three lists. These headings are also used in performance analysis to assess the levels of competence attained by the patient.

Applied analysis

This is meaningful only in relation to defined objectives and the assessed condition of the patient. Whether the therapist is selecting a single therapeutic activity or a range of options to offer the patient, or is seeking to modify the activity/task to make the performance of it possible, the content of the activity/task must first be analysed and evaluated using activity analysis, and then applied to the particular situation and the needs, interests and wishes of the individual by means of applied analysis. Aspects to consider might include, for example:

- patient's preferences and interests
- potential for engagement of patient interest and participation
- potential for choice or decision making
- potential for therapeutic adaptation to meet treatment objectives
- whether the activity is familiar to the patient — need for training or preparation in order to participate
- evaluation of whether or not the activity will meet the specified treatment objectives.

Selection of task for use as therapy. This may include:

- Select task which offers potential to achieve the therapeutic objective. Consider motor, sensory, interactive, cognitive, symbolic, expressive factors.
- Analyse task, breaking it into component parts: subtasks, skills, subskills. Decide which portions of the task have therapeutic value and require emphasis / are irrelevant or inappropriate / are to be done by the patient / should be done for the patient.
- Decide need for adaptation of tools, materials: identify need for preparation.

Activity synthesis

Combining components of the activity and environment to produce a desired therapeutic outcome.

Adaptation to activity

The activity may be presented in unadapted form or may be adapted to meet treatment goals. This is frequently tackled at the level of task adaptation since the adaptation required may differ from one stage of the activity to another. Typical adaptations are:

- *environmental*, e.g. location, setting, milieu; press
- *equipment*, e.g. quantity of tools / materials, adaptation to tools

- *social*, e.g. number of people, degree of interaction
- *physical*, e.g. position, strength, range of movement
- *cognitive*, e.g. complexity, sequence, need for instructions
- *emotional*, e.g. interest, meaning, self-expression
- *temporal*, e.g. duration, repetition
- *structural*, e.g. order of tasks, omission of non-essential tasks.

Grading

Manipulating factors required in the performance of a task or activity to meet treatment goals. Grading typically includes changes to:

- sequence of task / components
- size / shape of tools
- position of tools / furniture / materials
- quantity / specification of materials
- speed / duration / repetition of performance
- requirement for specific movements to perform task
- strength required
- perceptual components
- cognitive components
- simplicity / complexity
- type of / quantity of instruction / demonstration / sample
- the context (temporal, environmental, social, cultural) of the task
- the location and content of the environment in which the task is performed
- number of participants: requirement for interaction with others
- degree of choice / creativity / decision taking / planning and problem solving.

Environmental analysis and adaptation

This is another area of expertise unique to occupational therapists.

Content analysis

Occupational therapists recognize that the environment can have an important beneficial or detrimental effect on the individual. Analysis of the content of the environment—at work, at home, at school, in an institution, out of doors, in a public place—may provide information on the causes of problems for the individual, explanations for behaviour or ideas, or suggestions for therapeutic modifications.

> There is extensive discussion in the literature of the criteria for the selection or rejection of activities for use as therapy. Enduring arguments are:
>
> - Should OT only use purposeful, constructive activities? Are talking, thinking, imagining, relaxing, counselling, exercising, positioning, legitimate OT tools?
> - How far should activities be adapted—is there a risk of 'adapting the activity out of existence'?
> - The therapist often values the process above the product—but the reverse may be true of the patient. Can both be satisfied?
> - How directive should the therapist be in the selection of therapeutic activities? How much choice should the patient have?
>
> **Q** What is your opinion on the above questions? Make a few notes and then analyse what this indicates about your preferred model(s) and approach(es). Is your answer influenced by the nature of the client group with which you are working? Discuss your answers with others. Do you believe there are 'right' and 'wrong' answers?

Demand analysis

This is closely linked to content analysis and explores the psychological, cultural and social impact of the environment with reference to the effects of these factors in facilitating or inhibiting participation in occupations and activities.

The way in which environmental analysis is carried out depends on both the needs of the patient and the approach within which the therapist is working as these will alter the significance of the components which are observed.

In general terms, the occupational therapist will observe and acurately record environmental content—e.g. buildings, interiors, heat, light, sound, vibration, degree of stimulation, social or cultural significance, emotional impact—and define the environmental demand (syn. press) elements which contribute to or detract from patient performance.

Adaptation

The therapist may then alter, remove from or add to elements of the environment: e.g. physical features of buildings, access, sound, colour, lighting level, temperature, decor, furniture, information content, in order to remove obstacles to performance or to enhance the opportunities for performance, learning or development.

4

The philosophical and theoretical basis for practice

OPPOSING VIEWS OF REALITY

Before you tackle the literature on models and frames of reference it is important to recognize that there are two fundamentally different philosophical perspectives which underpin the various theories concerning the nature of human beings and their environment. These are alternative world views which are mutually incompatible; this does not mean that one is right and the other wrong (although some people do argue fervently for one view), merely that they are different explanations of objective and subjective reality. Many of the misunderstandings which arise when studying theoretical structures spring from a simple failure to take account of this dichotomy.

These perspectives are called the *reductionist* (atomist or mechanistic) point of view and the *holistic* (or organismic) point of view. These have been described as *metamodels* (Reed 1984) since all other models (or frames of reference) can be viewed as falling into one or other category, and I will use this term as a convenient shorthand (they can also be described as paradigms).

The terms given in brackets above are often used interchangeably, but they are not true synonyms, and the whole exercise of attempting to put models into neat pigeonholes is liable to oversimplfy some very complex philosophical arguments. Nonetheless, it may be helpful to have a basic understanding of the issues.

The reductionist generally takes an objective

and utilitarian view of concrete reality, which can be broken down into observable components. The whole may be understood by studying the parts. The universe operates by rules or laws which will, ultimately, be discovered.

The holist viewpoint is subjective; reality is mutable, the perceived world is indivisible; abstract and concrete elements interact and form a gestalt — a whole which is 'greater than the sum of its parts' — each element of which cannot be understood in isolation. This is also referred to as a *phenomenological* view of the world.

Linked with these opposing concepts is the ancient debate concerning free will and determinism. Is an individual able to make conscious and rational choices — a view held by most holistic philosophies — or are choices ultimately decided by factors such as environmental conditioning and the effects of past experience?

Another contentious area in philosophy is the argument between those who believe that human beings have both mind (and / or spirit) and body and that these are separate entities, a theory known as *dualism*, and those who believe that mind is inseparable from, or a product of, body, which is known as *monism*.

One can generally regard dualists as likely to take an holist standpoint and monists as taking a reductionist one—but some holistic philosophies believe strongly in the inseparability and close linkage between body and mind, and some mechanists simply disregard mind completely and only deal with body (and after that it really gets complicated!). If you wish to find out more about these ideas you will need to read books on metaphysics.

The main concepts of the two metamodels can be summarized (Box 4.1), but tempting though it is to make a nice neat list of opposites, it must be recognized that this involves simplification of highly complex debates and such generalization is inevitably not entirely accurate. A much more detailed discussion and comparison has been produced by Read (1984).

> **Q** Think about the differences in Box 4.1. How, in practical terms, does an awareness of the incompatibility of these metamodels help the therapist?

KEY SCHOOLS OF THOUGHT

Metamodels are of interest in the context of occupational therapy chiefly because it is agreed that occupational therapy is derived from an organismic, phenomenological view of the individual.

This raises the philosophical question of whether it is legitimate for occupational therapists to use reductionist frames of reference. Yet much of the foundation knowledge of occupational therapy is derived from the reductionist

---

Box 4.1 Comparison of holistic/organismic and reductionist/mechanistic metamodels

Holistic/organismic/phenomenological	Reductionist/mechanistic
Views person as a whole 'greater than the sum of its parts'.	Views individual as divisible into components which may be separately studied.
Tends to think of systems as interactive and adaptive.	Tends to think of systems as closed and fixed.
Control is based within the individual who has free will and can make conscious, rational decisions.	Deterministic: control is external to the individual, or has an involuntary basis.
Present/future oriented.	Past/present oriented.
Thoughts, feelings and perceptions are important and affect behaviour.	Behaviour is important: thoughts and emotions are by-products of physiology and/or behaviour.
Behaviour exceeds the utilitarian.	Behaviour is utilitarian.
Spirituality can be acknowledged.	Spirituality is not usually acknowledged.
Subjective methods of research are valid.	Objective methods are valid.

biological, behavioural and medical sciences. Occupational therapy's philosophy and practice have evolved from the application of such knowledge.

But occupational therapists also understand people from sociological and phenomenological perspectives; they are concerned with context and meaning and the subjective nature of experience. They are prepared to explore the significance of the symbolic and irrational aspects of human thought and behaviour. This seems to leave the profession uncomfortably straddling the great theoretical divide.

It is, therefore, useful briefly to review some key schools of thought, each of which produces a different theory of human behaviour. You will probably recognize these theories as the foundations of some widely used models or frames of reference in OT.

The key schools of thought providing explanations of behaviour can be summarized as follows:

- **Physiological**. We do what our genes and electrochemical functions make us capable of doing, in response to internal and external stimuli, to maintain homeostasis and satisfy basic needs.
- **Behavioural**. We perform and react as our environment demands in accordance with the consequences of such behaviour.
- **Cognitive**. We do what our thoughts and perceptions make us decide we should do.
- **Psychoanalytical**. We act in accordance with infantile drives and the unconscious memories of our pasts.
- **Developmental**. We develop the skills which time and opportunity have enabled us to gain.
- **Social**. We behave as we believe other people, specific social groups, or society as a whole, expect us to behave.
- **Humanistic**. We behave in accordance with our own choices, and in accordance with fundamental respect for others.
- **Systems theory**. We interact with our environment as part of an adaptive, organic, open system. We are shaped by our surroundings, and reciprocally shape other parts of the system.

Physiological and behavioural theories are based on the reductionist point of view. Research follows the principles of *scientific realism* or *logical empiricism*, in which reality is viewed as stable and measurable. These perspectives emphasize the necessity of objective studies under closely controlled experimental conditions, producing replicable results, in order to establish scientific principles, or facts about the human body or human behaviour. Such research is quantitative and is expected to produce statistics and carefully proven experimental data.

Psychoanalytical theories are also reductionist in that they stem from classical Freudian determinism — behaviour is influenced by unconscious drives and memories, past experiences and emotions, which can be analysed. However, the more recent holistic psychotherapeutic and humanist theories emphasize choice and free will and are holistic.

Cognitive, developmental, social, humanistic, and systems theories may be described as *organismic* and *phenomenological*. A phenomenological approach takes account of the subjective nature of experience and recognizes the unique and changing nature of this experience for each individual. In each of these theories the interaction of the person within the environment is important in different ways. Ecology is a recent influence in occupational therapy: from it is derived the concept of a person as an open system. In an open system (as opposed to a closed one which is fixed and non-responsive), the organism is responsive to its surroundings and behaves in a manner which both shapes the environment and is reciprocally shaped by it. The person can only be understood as part of a wider and more complex environment in which many organisms exist and interact.

Phenomenological research is more usually qualitative than quantitative and may use *ethnomethodological* techniques (derived from social anthropology), *naturalistic research* or *illuminative studies*. Use will be made of personal experience, descriptions, interviews, recordings, field studies and case studies which are typically hard to replicate and evaluate in strictly scientific terms. There is an increasing acceptance of the validity of the latter methods in the context of occupational therapy.

Why are these key schools of thought significant?

Humans are such complex organisms that more than one theory is needed to explain all the richness and intricacy of behaviour, thoughts and feelings. Having different perspectives can help the therapist to understand aspects of a person in differing ways and this may be helpful.

Too much may be made of 'the great divide'. However, you will probably have realized by now that combining techniques which are compatible with each other is likely to be more effective than trying to combine those from opposing perspectives.

For example, in its classical form, behaviourism is reductionist and deterministic. Humanism is holistic and self-actualizing. Using a rigid behavioural modification programme at the same time as a client centred programme emphasizing choice and self-actualization would be unlikely to work well as simultaneous treatments for an individual. (Conflicts of this kind are not unknown when different members of a treatment team work from the basis of incompatible models without adequate discussion.)

It is, therefore, important to be aware of the underlying philosophy of a model, frame of reference or approach and to ensure that the techniques used are compatible with it and each other. This is not to say that a skilful and experienced practitioner may not 'break the rules' and succeed in combining apparently incompatible techniques, but this should only be done deliberately and with caution.

Coping with the terminology

One of the chief difficulties for the student confronted by the literature on occupational therapy theory and struggling to obtain a clear concept of the meanings of various terms and their interrelationships is the realization that these change from one book to the next.

It is unfortunate that standard definitions of descriptive terms and concepts do not exist. British and American authors use terms in differing ways, and authors differ from each other. This is only partly due to differences between American English and British English, it is also due to differences in conceptualization. Words are frequently used loosely or interchangeably.

The words 'paradigm', 'model', 'frame of reference' and 'approach' are those which cause the most difficulty. Differing definitions abound and it is clear that we have still not reached a consensus within the profession about how these should be used.

Before we get tangled up in this debate, it is useful to explore what is meant by the words 'concept', 'hypothesis', 'theory' and 'philosophy' since on this at least there is agreement.

Concept

In psychology a *concept* is defined as 'The properties or relationships common to a class of objects or ideas', which may be abstract or concrete (Atkinson 1993).

A concept, then, is an idea which defines relationships and describes something. It is usually conveyed by words or a symbol of some kind. The 'conceptual foundations for practice' or 'concepts of occupational therapy' are the ideas which define what the profession is about, and which help to distinguish it from others.

Concepts are needed to build a body of knowledge and a good theory. A concept is an idea. If assumptions provide the foundations of a theory, then concepts provide the building blocks. As such the concepts can be organized into a framework that is systematic and interrelated and leads to the development of a theory (Reed and Sanderson 1992).

Hypothesis

'A proposition made as a basis for reasoning without assumption of its truth; a supposition made as a starting point for further investigation of known facts' (Concise Oxford Dictionary). A *hypothesis* is usually formulated with a view to testing it out by means of formal research; it may be proved or disproved, or may lead to the formulation of a new hypothesis.

As described in Chapter 5, generation and testing of hypotheses on an informal basis is an important part of clinical reasoning. Many theories incorporate hypotheses, some of which are so firmly established that they have become assumptions, i.e. statements which are accepted as true for the purposes of action.

Theory

'Supposition or system of ideas explaining something' is only the first of a number of definitions. This sounds at first rather like a concept, but a *theory* is a larger and more generalized entity which draws together concepts, hypotheses and assumptions to form a coherent explanation.

The theory sets out the explanation, it includes or assumes facts and phenomena, which may or may not be scientifically or objectively proved — the theory does not deal with such proof. 'The goal of theories is to create insights into nature' (Kielhofner 1995). Theories often bring with them statements about actions which can be taken on the assumption that the theory is true, and may indicate areas of research and associated methodology. The theory can be accepted as if it is true just so long as evidence exists which supports it, or until something has been done which disproves it.

This simple definition is misleading because it ignores the philosophical argument about the nature, purposes and validity of theory, systems for the construction of theories, and whether a theory can ever be proved or whether it can only be refuted. Theory building is itself subject to theory!

Different types of theories, and ways in which theories may be tested, are described, but this need not concern us here. Reed (1984) summarizes the main types of theory, or your librarian may suggest other books on theory building.

I will use theory as a convenient shorthand for all the ideas and concepts which provide the basis for professional practice.

Philosophy

The basic definition of *philosophy* is: 'seeking after wisdom or knowledge, especially that which deals with ultimate reality or with the most general causes and principles of things and ideas and human perception and knowledge of them' (Concise Oxford Dictionary).

When a profession's 'philosophy' is described, this means something rather different from the above definition. It implies a set of beliefs and ideas, the adoption of a particular 'world view', which the profession has accepted as a basis for academic and professional practice. The profession's principles, values and practice ought to be in accordance with its philosophy. It is generally accepted that occupational therapy has a holistic philosophy derived from the organismic meta-model.

Conflicting use of words

Discussion of the conceptual foundations for practice is relatively recent within occupational therapy, and both language and concepts are still being developed. Words tend to be borrowed from everyday speech or other sources and are then used in a sense particular to the context of occupational therapy, or as the author thinks best. The problem is that authors do not agree on usage. This may be intellectually exciting for those who like that sort of thing, but it is not helpful to the student who is trying to make sense of complex concepts.

It must sometimes seem as if the student is in a similar position to that of Alice in her famous exchange with Humpty Dumpty:

"There's glory for you!" "I don't know what you mean by 'glory'", Alice said, "I meant "There's a nice knock-down argument for you!" "But 'glory' doesn't mean 'a nice knock-down argument'" Alice objected. "When *I* use a word", Humpty Dumpty said in a rather scornful tone, "it means just what I choose it to mean – neither more nor less." (Lewis Carroll, *Alice Through the Looking Glass*)

The arguments over the use of the words paradigm, model, frame of reference and approach may be summarized as:

- Are these words synonyms, or do they have separate meanings?
- If they do have separate meanings, how should they be defined, how do they relate to each other, and which theories or concepts fit where in the taxonomy?
- Is the debate about words and meanings useful, or does it impede our ability to understand how theory is put into practice (i.e. do the words really matter)?

I will explore each of these questions with reference to current opinions.

Synonyms or not?

As already noted, the words used to describe occupational therapy theory are used loosely and apparently interchangeably.

The degree of confusion which still prevails is best illustrated by comparing the ways in which recent OT textbooks use the words which describe theory.

It seems that in practice these words *are* used to some extent as synonyms. It is also clear that allocation of the various kinds of 'models' to each classification is quite arbitrary.

The fact that the words are used interchangeably in this way does not, however, mean that they *are* synonyms; it may simply indicate that the terminology of model building is in a developmental stage, and that there is a degree of confusion and disagreement concerning the appropriate use of the words. Certainly there is no one formula for terminology or classification.

Confusion over the word *paradigm* is understandable, since different authorities define it differently, and one influential scientific author — Kuhn — gives several versions of his own view. There is also disagreement over whether or not occupational therapy possesses a defined paradigm. The majority view is probably that it is still developing one, or that there are several variations.

Creek (1990) proposed an OT paradigm. She defines the term as: 'An agreed body of theory explaining and rationalizing professional unity and practice, that incorporates all the profes-

sion's concerns, concepts and expertise and guides values and commitments.' Another version (Kielhofner 1988) states that it is: 'A consensus of the most fundamental beliefs or assumptions of a field.'

Whether or not the profession has yet achieved a paradigm, there are several definitions of OT which share the common theme of the importance of occupations in promoting and sustaining healthy and meaningful human life and their potential use as therapy. It may be that an OT paradigm, if or when eventually decided, will relate to these fundamental elements of the profession.

Debates over the difference between *model* and *frame of reference* and the relationship between these (if any) can quickly become as convoluted and impenetrable as the medieval clerics' discussion of the number of angels able to dance on the head of a pin. The following quotations provide you with a sample:

In summary, model building is composed of five phases which form a sequence of interlocking systems … the frame of reference, assumptions and concepts are crucial to exploring, organizing and developing the model…. [a frame of reference is] a mechanism which can be used to explain the relationship of theory to action … [it] is not the total model but does form part of the model building process (Reed 1984).

Although professions have only one Model they usually have a variety of frames of reference … [which] derive from a profession's model, provide guidance on day to day interaction with clients. A frame of reference is far more limited than a model (Mosey 1986).

A frame of reference refers to principles behind practice with a specific patient or client population. It includes a statement of the population to be served, guidelines for determining adequate function or dysfunction and principles for remediation (Bruce & Borg 1987).

Within each frame of reference, one or more models has developed to give more specific direction to practice in the various areas in which occupational therapists work (Creek 1990).

I stress that conceptual models of practice make theoretical arguments; Mosey notes that frames of reference only create applications of existing theory. Conceptual models of practice address a particular component of occupational behaviour or motivation

Table 4.1   Comparisons of terminology used to describe theory: American sources

Source	Paradigm	Model	Frame of reference
Reed (1984)	Discussed in detail; Not the same as model or theory, both 'may be contained within a paradigm.' Explains phenomena; comprehensive; new ideas; ideas for research.	Describes model building in detail. 'conceptual or theoretical models are subtype . . . which relate to theory building and explanation . . . . Reed provides list of models too long to quote.	Gives various definitions. 'involves a mechanism which leads to development and use of a standard, schema or set of facts to judge, control or direct some action or expression.' 'A frame of reference is not a model but does form part of the model building process . . . it explains the relationship of theory to action.'
Mosey (1986)	(Philosophical assumptions and Model) Does not use term *paradigm*.	(see paradigm) 'defines and delineates the broad outlines of the profession'	'delineates a particular area or aspect (of OT) – links model and practice' Analytical Developmental (Recapitulation of ontogenesis) Acquisitional
Kielhofner (1992)	Paradigm 'Core assumptions; focal viewpoint; values → fundamental nature and purpose of OT'	Conceptual practice models. 'presents and organizes theoretical concepts used by OTs; expresses theory unique to OT' Biomechanical Cognitive disabilities Cognitive perceptual Group work Model of human occupation Motor control (e.g. Bobath, PNF) Sensory integration Spatiotemporal adaptation	
Willard & Spackman 8th edn. (1993)	Paradigm (discussed as one name for 'intervening mechanism between theory and practice')	synonym for paradigm (as Mosey)	defined as Mosey 'four hierarchical components: theoretical base; function-dysfunction continuum; behaviours indicative of function/dysfunction; postulates regarding change' Behavioural Biomechanical Cognitive disability Developmental Neurodevelopmental Sensory integration Model of human occupation Rehabilitation Psychodynamic Spatiotemporal adaptation Occupational adaptation

Table 4.2 Comparisons of terminology used to describe theory: British sources

Source	Paradigm	Model	Frame of reference	Approach
Young & Quinn (1992)	Discusses scientific origins of term but does not describe an 'OT paradigm'. Describes a 'hard core' of OT knowledge with a 'protective belt' of optional, useful theories.	Function of model: 'framework for complex data; visualization of phenomena; communication of ideas; predictions about real world; stimulates development of theories.'	Functions: 'It specifies the nature, aims and procedures of the work and the features which distinguish it from other forms of practice; it suggests that some theories are more relevant to practice than others.' Adaptive performance Developmental Sensorimotor Cognitive Role performance Rehabilitation	
Turner (1992)	Describes philosophy and values. 'A paradigm imposes shape upon a science. It derives from profession's shared values, principles and knowledge and determines the scope and boundaries of the profession, guiding practice, research and development.' 'provides a general structure for thought'	'Conceptual model represents basic theories behind practice, delineating the framework for action ... and displays links between theory and practice.' Model of human occupation Developmental Occupational performance	'organized body of knowledge, principles and research findings which forms the conceptual basis of a particular aspect of practice — explains relationship between theory and practice' Humanistic Mosey's 3 F of R (see Table 3.1) Biomechanical Compensatory (Rehab) Learning	'ways and means of doing, i.e. implementing frames of reference'
Creek (1992)	Proposes OT paradigm 'an agreed body of theory explaining and rationalizing professional unity and practice ... incorporates all the profession's concerns, concepts and expertise, and guides values and commitment.'	'Simplified representation of structure and content ... that describes or explains complex relationships between concepts.' Activities therapy Communication Developmental Model of human occupation	'The principles behind practice; the organization of knowledge in a particular field to permit description of the relationships between facts and concepts.' Psychodynamic Behavioural Developmental Humanistic Adaptive performance Biodevelopment Developmental Occupational behaviour	

(e.g. motivation, movement, perception, sensory integration) and seek to explain how this aspect of occupation is organized .... they also seek to explain states of disorder or dysfunction. In addition [they] result in clinical technology. Finally, they generate a research base (Kielhofner 1992).

Frames of reference are derived from a profession's

model, but they are narrower in focus and different in intent (Willard & Spackman 1994).

In these circumstances, confusion in the mind of the student is legitimate and one can only sympathize with authors who invent their own terminology: 'We use the terms 'theoretical framework' and 'theory' in this paper to connote 'theory', 'model' and 'theoretical approach' because the latter terms have no accepted definitions in the profession' (Javatz & Katz 1989).

One has to wade through this muddy bog of words in order to reach the firm ground of the concepts which underlie them.

It is plain from a more detailed analysis of the literature that most American authors fall into one of two 'camps' when they discuss theory. Those who follow Mosey use the term 'frame of reference' to describe the theoretical structures which occupational therapists use to guide practice, and 'OT model' to mean a statement of the fundamental principles and practice of the profession. Those who follow Keilhofner and his associates prefer the term 'model' for the former and 'paradigm' for the latter, however, the basic concepts which each are trying to describe are fundamentally similar.

In Britain, where influence from both camps has been combined with traditional English usage, including the word 'approach', authors tend to put forward their personal interpretations of terminology and the relationship between these concepts.

Kortman (Australia) (1994), having analysed current usage, dismisses the semantic debate as follows:

The fact that there are so many definitions with so little agreement between theorists suggests that theorists are taking the wrong path by trying to constantly redefine terms.

He concludes straightforwardly that the words are synonyms:

Put simply, in common English, a model is a frame of reference is a paradigm is an approach; the terms are interchangeable. Of all these the term model appears to be the simplest to use in relation to theory.

It would be fine, and a relief to all concerned, if it was as simple as this, however, Kortman then has to accept that 'models are not uniform in type' and finds it necessary to describe three different types of model, arranged as an hierarchy: *professional model* (i.e. paradigm/OT model); *delineation model* (i.e. frame of reference/model); and *application model* (i.e. approach) thus somewhat weakening his argument.

The point that he is making is, nonetheless, important; understanding what models et al are *for* may be a better way of sorting out the language than involved semantic debates.

For the present, therefore, let us ignore the terminology and concentrate on the underlying concepts concerning the different functions of theory.

Basic concepts

Six basic concepts concerning the theoretical foundations of the profession are found in most texts.

Concept 1: 'The grand design'

The need for an overview which defines the nature of occupational therapy as a profession.

Its purpose is to give a description of what OT is, its philosophy, principles, assumptions, values, and beliefs, and the nature of its practice (and, by exclusion, defines what it is not, and what it does not do).

Concept 2: 'Borrowed knowledge'

Concept 2 can be subdivided into two closely related forms of 'borrowing'.

Concept 2a: 'Borrowed science'. The need to use basic sciences (e.g. anatomy, psychology, sociology, health sciences) as appropriate to the context of OT practice.

Its purpose is to provide useful explanations of function and dysfunction and the scientific basis for and justification of practice.

Concept 2b: 'Borrowed skills'. The need to learn skills developed by others (e.g. teaching; counselling; group therapy) with the related theories.

The purpose here is to provide the therapist with a repertoire of skills which will be useful in treating occupational dysfunction.

Concept 3: 'The OT version'

The need to apply and adapt elements drawn from relevant theory, together with appropriate skills in the context of occupational therapy for a specific speciality.

Its purpose is to help the individual OT to develop and use a repertoire of therapy and other interventions within a coherent and consistent theoretical framework when working with individuals or groups. It provides a well defined basis for practice and aids clinical reasoning.

Concept 4: 'Pure OT'

The need for therapists to construct widely applicable systems of theory and practice in relation to the core principles, knowledge and values of OT, as distinct from those 'borrowed' from other professions.

The purpose here is to simplify, explain, organize and synthesize knowledge relevant to OT and relate this to practice. It provides impetus for research and the further development of OT theory and aids clinical reasoning.

Concept 5: 'Making it work'

The need to put theory into practice.

It provides the therapist with a repertoire of appropriate and compatible, methodology, assessments or techniques.

Concept 6: 'Processes of change'

These are somewhat different from the others. There are four models/frames of reference which have been very influential in OT theory building and practice, and which are frequently referred to in texts, but which fail to fit neatly into any of the concepts just described.

Sometimes these are also referred to as processes—means whereby an individual is sequentially changed over the passage of time. These are:

Development. The natural processes of change between infancy and adulthood.

Education. A process which results in learning—'The relatively permanent changes in potential for performance that results from past interactions with the environment' Lovell (1987).

Rehabilitation. Structured change leading to recovery from illness or injury.

Adaptation. Change which is useful to the individual and which promotes health, well-being and survivial.

The problem is that each of these processes is so large and important in its own right that it operates at various levels and can be viewed as fitting with Concepts 1, 2, 3, and 5, and influencing the development of 'pure OT' models, Concept 4.

These processes of change will be discussed in more detail in Section 3 and I will leave Concept 6 out of the analysis for the time being.

Overlapping terminology

As shown in the previous quotations and Table 4.1, terms are used as synonyms to identify these concepts. This overlapping use of terminology to define the five concepts given above (excluding concept 6) is shown in Box 4.2.

Summary

So, has this complex discussion of language enabled us to reach any conclusions?

The answer to the question 'are the terms synonyms?' seems to be:

yes, they are used as synonyms
but
the concepts which they attempt to describe are not the same.

My personal conclusion is that distinct concepts ought to have different names by which they can be distinguished from each other, and that continued use of available terminology as if it was totally interchangeable is not helpful.

The problem is that we have still not reached a consensus as to which terms should be used to indicate which concepts. Should we decide to use existing terminology in a particular way, or should we, as Kortman suggests, adopt a new descriptive structure?

Since for practical purposes we must continue to use the language we have until a better taxonomy is evolved, it seems important to ensure that terms are used in a way which is clear, logical, well defined and consistent.

Box 4.2				
Concept 1: **The grand** **design**	**Concept 2:** **Borrowed** **knowledge**	**Concept 3:** **The OT** **version**	**Concept 4:** **Pure** **OT**	**Concept 5:** **Making it** **work**
OT model	Theory	Frame of reference	Frame of reference	Frame of reference
Paradigm	Frame of reference	Conceptual practice Model	OT model	Model
Core principles	Basic science	Model	Generic model	Approach
Professional model	Conceptual framework	Delineation model		Application model

DEFINITIONS OF TERMINOLOGY AS USED IN THIS BOOK

An attempt to find a unifying definition for each term at this stage is probably either brave or foolhardy, but I cannot write this book on the basis of continual 'ifs and buts', and since I have an aversion to imprecise use of language in an academic context, I must make some decisions. Let us begin with some general definitions.

Paradigm

The paradigm consists of the basic assumptions, values and perspectives that unify the field. It defines and gives coherence or wholeness to the entire profession. It speaks to the nature and purpose of occupational therapy. It gives therapists a common understanding of what it means to be an occupational therapist (Kielhofner 1992) (syn. Professional model).

A paradigm or professional model gives an overview of what the profession is concerned with, and what its practitioners do (and do not) do. It is the overall plan or template for occupational therapy as a whole (Concept 1: The grand design).

In its scientific meaning, a paradigm is a rather rigid entity which does not evolve but is replaced at intervals by a new paradigm. The OT paradigm does not appear to me to be of this type; it is more like a general pattern for the profession. The core concepts do not change, but there is room for evolution and development so that practice can adapt to meet the changing needs of health care and society as a whole.

I prefer to use *paradigm* istead of its synonym *professional model* as the distinct word helps to emphasize that it is different in content and scope from OT practice models.

Models

A simplified representation of structure and content of a phenomenon or system that describes or explains complex relationships between concepts within the system and integrates elements of theory and practice.

The key words in this definition are 'simplified', 'describes', 'explains', and 'integrates theory and practice'. A model ought to make things simpler to understand. It takes several different elements, shows the relationships between them, and makes them into a unified whole. It also gives guidance on what to do.

An OT practice model tends to be related closely to the paradigm / professional model, and gives general guidance on the practice of occupational therapy, usually applicable to all types of patients or to a wide group (e.g. psychosocial dysfunction) (Concept 4: Pure OT).

Frames of reference

A system of theories serving to orient or give meaning to a set of circumstances which provides a coherent conceptual basis for therapy.

The problem with this term is that it has been used in two different but related ways.

In the first sense the term is used to indicate theory relevant to occupational therapy which has been taken from various basic sciences. This is how Kielhofner (1992) uses the word, i.e. to convey Concept 2: Borrowed knowledge. I will continue to use primary frame of reference (PFR) in this sense.

In the second sense, as used for example by Dutton, Levy and Simon (Hopkins & Smith [Willard & Spackman] 1994), it means a version of theory adapted and applied for OT practice, i.e. Concept 3: The OT Version and/or Concept 5: Approach (thus producing a tautology such as 'the model of human occupation frame of reference'). Using the same word for two different concepts is confusing, so I will use the term applied frame of reference (AFR) to describe application within OT specialities of theories derived from outside the profession.

Approaches

Ways and means of putting theory into practice (Concept 5: Making it work).

An approach is often connected with an applied frame of reference, and gives techniques, assessments or procedures which are useful when carrying out treatment in a particular setting with a particular client group. It deals with practical aspects of what to do, not with the theory behind the 'doing', which is expressed in the AFR.

Confusion can be caused because approaches sometimes have the same name as the applied frame of reference from which they are derived. For example, the behavioural frame of reference (psychological/learning theory) gives rise to an applied frame of reference, also called behavioural (describing how behavioural theory applies to OT) and to a behavioural modification approach (describing behavioural assessments and techniques).

OT models may also generate approaches, but more often they utilize a variety of approaches drawn from several applied frames of reference.

One needs some criteria by which to decide whether or not one is justified in calling a style of practice an approach. My own test is that an approach should:

- **Have boundaries to the content:** possess a

definable and coherent set of concepts which are distinctly different from other sets.
- **Be directive and exclusive:** oblige one to think and act in a circumscribed manner when working within it, excluding ideas and actions which are incompatible or irrelevant.
- **Enable a clear definition of the patient/ client's problem to be made:** provide an explanation for the origin of the client's dysfunction or need, and consequent guidance on appropriate action.
- **Have defined methods of practical application:** provide one with a related set of assessment and treatment techniques which are used in a specific way within it.
- **Include a unique definition of outcome**: enable the practitioner to judge success or failure within the context of the approach.

PROCESSES OF CHANGE

Means whereby an individual sequentially changes over the passage of time in ways which are beneficial to his health, well-being, and ability to survive. These processes include: development, education, rehabilitation, adaptation (see Section 3).

Box 4.3 summarizes the concepts and related terms used in this book.

Box 4.3 Concepts and terms used in this book	
Concept	**Term**
Concept 1: The grand design	Paradigm (syn. Professional model)
Concept 2: Borrowed knowledge Borrowed skill	Primary frame of reference
Concept 3: The OT version	Applied frame of reference
Concept 4: Pure OT	OT practice model
Concept 5: Making it work	Approach
Concept 6: Processes of change	Processes of change

More comprehensive definitions for each term are given in the Glossary (p. 141)

Relationships between the concepts

It is tempting to arrange these concepts as an hierarchy, moving from theory towards practice. This is what Kortman (1994) has suggested.

The relationship is not, in my view, a simple linear one, for there are more complex relationships and interactions between the concepts (Fig. 4.1).

The theories which underpin basic sciences, frames of reference and processes of change are all derived from sources external to occupational therapy. Selected elements from these theories and associated practices find their way into the OT paradigm, which also includes theory developed by and unique to the profession.

Frames of reference are adapted by occupational therapists to form applied frames of reference, and these in turn lead to the development of approaches which includes styles of relationship between OT and patient, means of assessment or evaluation and means of treating, or intervening on behalf of, the patient.

The OT paradigm and processes of change form the background to OT models, which then utilize approaches derived from compatible frames of reference to provide a wide range of treatment techniques. Sometimes the OT Model generates its own approach.

As practice evolves and develops, information is fed back into the OT paradigm, parts of which may thereby change and evolve, although this process is slow, and the fundamental principles are not affected.

WHICH STRUCTURES FOR PRACTICE FIT WHERE?

Having decided on definitions, it may seem that the problems of deciding which theory fits where—whether it is part of the profession's paradigm or whether it is a model or a frame of reference—would be relatively simple. Unfortunately, this is not so, for our conceptualization of the profession and its practice has not yet unravelled these relationships. The individual author must still choose her own logical structure for such allocation.

The classification system which I use is my

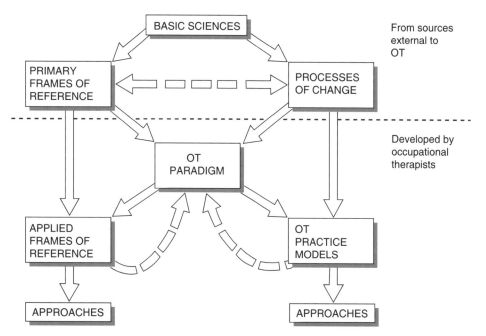

Figure 4.1   Relationships between the concepts.

Box 4.4 Are you still muddled about the use and meaning of these terms?

If you are, do not worry—you can understand the rest of this book without needing to be too precise about the distinctions between terms, and your understanding of them will probably become clearer as you read on. If you disagree with me and have become used to different definitions, stick with them for the moment and review whether you wish to change your views later.

It may help you to relate the terms to a more familiar concept: that of designing a house.

You start with a general concept of a house: it must have a floor, roof, walls and various rooms. You may choose to include the ideas of an apartment or bungalow in your definition, but you will probably decide that a tent or a caravan are not 'houses' in the usual sense of the word.

This is your **paradigm**. It tells you what OT is about and helps you to decide what is, or is not, OT.

A house may contain various rooms—kitchen; bathroom; living-room; cellar; attic; nursery; etc. Each contains different furniture and appliances and has a different purpose. Some of the above rooms will be useful to you, others may not.

The rooms are your **Applied frames of reference**. You can choose to use the ones which are appropriate.

Now you can design a particular **kind** of house: you will select a size and shape suited to your special purposes, and will choose to include certain rooms and to leave others out.

This is your **OT model**. It brings certain ideas together and excludes others.

Finally, you can move into your house and start to live there. At certain times you may use one room and its contents; at others you may move around using different rooms or parts of a room or the appliances within it. However, you can only use what is in the house.

This is your **approach**. You can choose which techniques or media to use, but you can only use the ones which are available within the model or frame of reference you are working with.

---

personal system of conceptualization and therefore requires some explanation and justification. There is an important distinction between the organizational model which I present, which you may choose to accept or reject, and the description of each theoretical structure which attempts to present an objective summary of currently accepted thinking. An organizational structure for terms classifying different things is called a taxonomy.

Taxonomy of frames of reference, models and approaches

The classification system used in this book is divided as follows: Section 2 deals with primary frames of reference (PFR) which offer differing perspectives on human function and dysfunction, and their associated applied frames of reference (AFR) and approaches. The justification for inclusion in this section is that practice is based mainly on theories or skills which have originat-ed from sources outside the profession. These are shown in Box 4.5.

Processes of change are described in Chapter 9 which deals with development, education, rehabilitation and adaptation and also describes a problem based process model by which these four processes may be integrated.

OT practice models are described in Chapter 10. The rationale for inclusion is that these are models created by occupational therapists which synthesize theories and practices from various sources from a uniquely OT perspective, with an emphasis on the occupational nature of human beings.

- Adaptive skills and recapitulation of ontogenesis (Mosey)
- Adaptation through occupation (Reed)
- Model of human occupation (Keilhofner)
- Cognitive disabilities (Alan)
- Occupational performance and the client centred model for practice (Law et al Canadian OTA)

Box 4.5   Frames of reference and approaches

Primary frame of reference	Applied frame of reference	Approaches
Physiological	Biomechanical	Biomechanical Activities of daily living Compensatory
	Neurodevelopmental	Bobath Pnf Rood Conductive education (Peto)
	Sensory integration	Sensory integration (Ayres) Sensory integration (King)
Psychology	Behavioural	Behavioural modification
	Cognitive	Cognitive-perceptual Cognitive-behavioural
Psychiatry and psychotherapy	Psychodynamic	Analytical group work communication
Humanism	Humanistic	Client centred Student centred learning

Do the words matter?

At one level, the answer is no. The student or practitioner need not get involved in the debates over terminology, provided that he or she understands that there are different concepts and levels of conceptualization when it comes to describing theory.

It *is* important to use the language consistently, either selecting one system and sticking to it, or using the language appropriate to the theorist whose ideas or model you are using.

It is also important to understand that there are a range of models or frames of reference to guide practice. If the language gets in the way, ignore it — but do not ignore the ideas which it is trying to convey.

At another level, that of the academic and intellectual development of the profession, terminology and taxonomy are important, because they contribute to theory building and to the description of the scientific basis for practice.

It is important, however, that the profession does not allow itself to become sidetracked into semantic debate instead of paying attention to the real issues of developing a coherent and comprehensible theoretical foundation for practice.

5

Linking theory with practice

WHY USE A THEORETICAL STRUCTURE?

Using an applied frame of reference or model provides you with the mental equivalent of a map to guide the treatment process. This is helpful to the student who needs a framework within which to work. It helps to limit possibilities and to focus the mind in a particular direction. Correctly used it will help you to make good therapeutic decisions by offering a coherent framework for practice relevant to the needs of the patient. It may aid multidisciplinary communication by clarifying expectations and the basis for therapy. For the more experienced practitioner, a theoretical structure provides a rationale for practice, a basis for research or reflection, and an analytical tool.

By now it should be clear that there are many available structures for practice. How does one avoid becoming totally bewildered and how does one choose the right one for any given situation?

Ways of using theory

Theory is built into the OT paradigm, part of 'the core', and the competent practitioner ought to be firmly grounded in that knowledge and able to use it to explain and justify practice.

But each individual patient presents a new situation; a selection needs to be made from the available theories which fit the case. If you study representations of the OT process, it soon becomes clear that authors have two views of when this should take place. Some describe the selection of a model or AFR as happening at the very start of the process, before any information has been collected. Others describe a process of information gathering and analysis which leads to the selection of a suitable approach. There are also two ways of describing the use of theoretical structures, as a conceptual lens (Kielhofner 1992) and as a tool. These two points of selection and two different metaphors are linked, and each indicates a different way of using theory, so it is worth exploring these distinctions further.

A conceptual lens

If you take up a lens, or put on a pair of coloured spectacles, you immediately change what you are looking at. What you see is in some way coloured, filtered or focused by the lens.

If you use a theoretical framework — an applied frame of reference or an OT model — as a 'lens', you select it right at the start of the process. You 'put on the spectacles' before you ever encounter a patient. You then look at the patient and his problems through that lens, and this changes what you see and how you interpret it.

In some situations the therapist will choose to use one particular applied frame of reference or OT model and no other. For example, you may choose to work in a department, unit or area which deals with one client group or speciality, where the staff already have a clear idea of the approach they wish to use and everyone follows this, e.g. a psychotherapeutic unit using a particular analytical theory, a neurological unit using a neurodevelopmental technique, or an orthopaedic unit using a biomechanical approach.

Alternatively, you may make a personal decision to adopt a particular applied frame of reference or a more broadly based OT model, such as the model of human occupation.

When the patient is referred, the therapist can use the language and techniques of the approach and interpret the patient's problems, and plan consequent actions, in accordance with the chosen structure. In this way practice is *theory driven*. (See Fig. 5.1.)

Sometimes theory which is used in this way becomes so integrated with practice that it almost disappears — at least the practitioners cease to be aware of using it. Probably the emphasis is so firmly on the approach, the 'doing' aspects, that the theory gets pushed into the background. A little 'excavation' will usually enable the therapist to track back from what was done to the underlying rationale provided by the theory.

A tool

If you work in the community, or in any area where you have a wide range of patients, the theory driven pattern may be too restrictive. You need to use a wide range of approaches, dependent on the type of problem which the patient has.

You can use the OT process to gather information in order to name the problem and decide how to frame it. You can then decide which of the available approaches you want to use as a 'tool' on this occasion, set goals and choose techniques. In this case you are being *process driven* — using the structure of the OT process to define the patient's needs and direct what you do.

Of course, you need to choose the right 'tool' for the task; sometimes there is a wide choice and sometimes a narrow one. If you need to knock in a nail you automatically pick a hammer, not a screwdriver, but to drill a hole you can choose from a hand-drill, brace and bit, bradawl, auger, electric drill or pillar drill. This may seem confusing, but only if you are not a carpenter, to whom the choice would be obvious. Similarly, if you are using the process driven pattern, the selection of an appropriate approach becomes easier when you have expertise as a therapist. (See Fig. 5.2.)

Other considerations

These two patterns of practice are alternatives which are suited to different situations.

It is important to retain flexibility, especially if using a specific frame of reference. Nothing can be gained by artificially trying to 'fit the patient to the theory'. You must always question whether the chosen structure really does match the patient's needs. It is quite possible to move from being theory driven to being process driven and back again if required. A therapist who only knows a few approaches would be very limited and would need to retrain if moving into a different speciality.

Selection of a structure also depends on your personal knowledge and expertise: this may be limited with regard to the use of some specialist approaches or techniques, or your personal style may make you more comfortable with some than with others.

Some approaches require considerable experience and expertise. We all have to start somewhere but it is not wise to attempt to use a technique which you only partly understand

unless you have found someone experienced to give you close supervision until you become proficient.

Are theoretical structures really necessary?

It is, arguably, perfectly possible to be a good therapist without ever consciously using a model or frame of reference, provided that your core skills are well developed (although the theory is there somewhere if you start to look for it). You would, however, miss out on much valuable information.

It is equally possible to know a great deal about theory and to remain an indifferent thera-

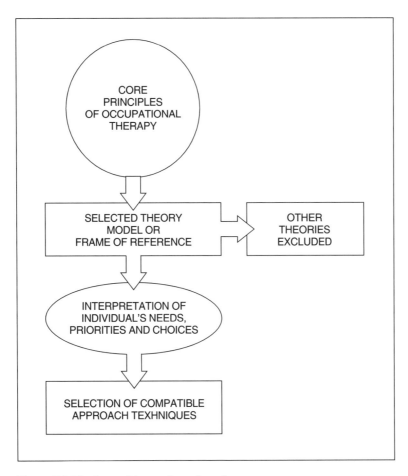

Figure 5.1 The theory driven pattern of practice.

pist. The lens is only as good as the trained perceptions of the user; the tool is only as good as the skill and understanding of the craftsman — and we all know that 'bad workmen blame their tools'.

The skill of selecting and using structures for practice is closely linked with the skills of clinical reasoning which provide the cognitive basis for effective practice. The modes of clinical reasoning used by therapists will be described in the next section.

CLINICAL REASONING

Clinical reasoning describes the cognitive processing used by a health care professional when making judgements and decisions concerning a patient. These reasoning processes have been studied in doctors, nurses, and other professionals and, more recently, in occupational therapists.

Clinical reasoning can be defined as:

The process of systematic decision making based on an identifiable professional frame of reference (i.e. applied frame of reference or OT model) and utilizing both subjective and objective data accrued through appropriate assessment / evaluation processes (Willard and Spackman 1994).

Burke and De Poy (1991) write:

An understanding of the clinical reasoning process may reveal the unique ways that occupational therapists come to assess and seek solutions to

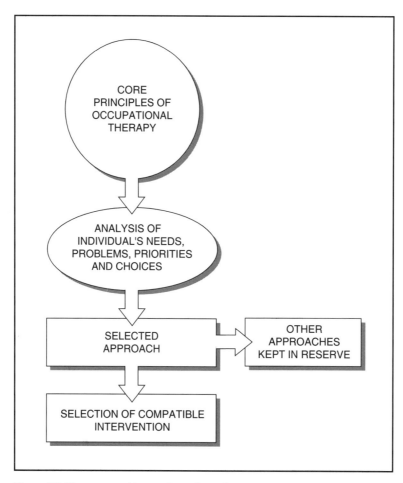

Figure 5.2 The process driven pattern of practice.

patients' problems and to delimit the scope of their practice to what is uniquely occupational therapy. Clinical reasoning addresses many of the unstated thoughts and formulations that therapists develop when they work with patients.

There are some important points in this passage: clinical reasoning involves the cognition which underlies the process of naming, framing and problem solving; secondly, and even more fundamentally, it concerns the cognitive patterns which translate the knowledge, skills and values of the therapist into action and which ensure that occupational therapists practice occupational therapy, and not some other form of intervention. Thirdly, it involves thinking which is complex, often so rapid that it seems 'intuitive', and by its very nature hard to capture and describe.

Therapists are people; they process information and make judgements and decisions like all other human beings. Secondly, they are health care professionals, they share elements of the knowledge and skills which are common to all these professions, and they think in ways which are basically similar to doctors or nurses or other professionals. Thirdly, they are occupational therapists who have a unique body of knowledge and practice which influences the conclusions they reach and the actions they take.

The occupational therapy process provides the organizing structure for practice, but as already noted it is not unique to occupational therapy. It is the use of clinical reasoning which results in occupational therapy.

Once you have learnt to 'think like a therapist' you go on 'thinking like a therapist' and, although you may be given the same set of facts about a patient as the doctor or the nurse, the physiotherapist or the social worker, the way you describe the problems and the actions you take ought to be different. Because you have learnt the knowledge and skills of an occupational therapist, and because you understand the nature of occupational therapy and its core concerns and practices, even though you are using the same mental mechanisms as other health workers, you will think and act like an occupational therapist, and not like a doctor or a nurse.

Of course in practice the roles of various professions merge and overlap, but it is important for occupational therapy as a profession, and for its effectiveness as a therapy, that the unique focus of the profession is not submerged by multidisciplinary practice. Well developed clinical reasoning enables the therapist to maintain this clear focus.

The study of clinical reasoning in occupational therapy is relatively recent and the terminology is still developing — indeed, in this respect, it is rather like the study of theoretical structures. It can become confusing reading various books and papers when you discover that (by now you will not be surprised!) similar terms are used by different authors to mean different things. The student needs to remember that this literature is based on a relatively small number of influential studies, mostly in America, and she must try to see past the rather confusing terminology to the basic concepts which are being described.

Reasoning modes

There does seem to be agreement that OTs use several different reasoning modes. Fleming (1991 and Mattingly & Fleming 1994) has described 'three track reasoning'. Some of these reasoning modes are similar to those identified in studies of medical reasoning and are quite well understood, other modes have been proposed as distinctly characteristic of occupational therapists.

Box 5.1 summarizes, in simplified form, the main reasoning modes which have been described to date. If you are interested in finding out more about clinical reasoning, you will need to refer to the texts listed at the end of this chapter.

Cognitive processes

Effective clinical reasoning depends on the use of some basic cognitive processes, so it may be helpful to summarize these.

Cognitive processes are defined as 'Mental processes of perception, memory and informa-

---

Box 5.1 Modes of clinical reasoning

Reasoning mode	Purpose
Diagnostic reasoning	To identify functional problems towards which occupational therapy will be directed; to make problem statements about occupational performance; to define desired outcomes, set goals and develop solutions. Diagnostic reasoning employs the four stage model of hypothetical reasoning: cue acquisition and pattern recognition; hypothesis generation; cue evaluation; hypothesis testing (Rogers & Holm 1991).
Predictive reasoning	During predictive reasoning the therapist weighs probabilities and possibilities and attempts to predict the effects of options for intervention and to gain a picture of probable outcomes in the case in relation to various imagined scenarios (Hagedorn 1995b).
Procedural reasoning	To select solutions, procedures and actions which the therapist and/or patient may use to achieve the desired outcome, or any associated objective. Procedural reasoning gives the experienced therapist rapid access to appropriate, automated patterns of action and interaction (Fleming 1994).
Pragmatic reasoning	In its simpler form this mode addresses the practicalities of therapy — evaluation of whether an action is feasible, and whether the context and resources in a given situation facilitate an intervention or make it inadvisable. It has also been suggested (Rogers & Holm 1991) that it also takes account of the therapist's knowledge, skill, and interests and wider organizational, sociocultural and political considerations.
Ethical reasoning	Through ethical reasoning the therapist evaluates proposed interventions in relation to the moral and ethical basis of practice, and with regard to any medicolegal considerations. There are clear guidelines on ethical practice which all therapists must follow. Ethical reasoning becomes especially important in situations where the patient is vulnerable and unable to express personal wishes.
Interactive reasoning	As proposed by Fleming (1994), this takes place during therapeutic use of self to modify the therapist's approach in response to what the patient says or the non-verbal signals he produces. The therapist uses interactive reasoning to gain rapport, to promote trust, to motivate the patient, and to gain empathetic understanding of him as a person.
Narrative reasoning	As proposed by Mattingly (1994) this involves the use of clinical story-telling either as an aid to understanding the patient and planning therapy, or as an aid to reflective practice by analysing the informal stories which therapists tell each other when describing practice.

---

tion processing by which the individual acquires information, makes plans and solves problems' (Atkinson 1993).

The phrase 'acquires information, makes plans and solves problems' is a reasonable summary of what the occupational therapist does when planning and initiating an intervention, a process in which the major part of the therapist's actions may often be 'thinking in order to do', rather than actual 'doing'.

This definition therefore highlights the main mental processes involved — perception, memory and information processing — and the skill components of these processes. These in turn are associated with, and developed through, learning and experience.

The information processing model of cognition involves input, coding, storage and retrieval. Input is crucial, for if information is not attended to and coded correctly it cannot be stored or retrieved.

Information may be processed in serial form, only one source being attended to at a time, or in parallel, in which several sources of information can be dealt with simultaneously. Some forms of processing are automatic and used unconsciously, others require attention.

Pattern recognition

In order to recognize a pattern the observer must use the sequence of observe pattern → identify cues → determine pattern → relate to type. Much of the research into pattern recognition has been focused on visual perception, however, the principles can be extended to wider contexts. People tend to perceive stimuli according to factors such as proximity, similarity and closure (perceptual patterning) and impose organization on any perceived pattern in order to see it as a whole (gestalt).

Pattern recognition requires attention, the conscious focusing of perception on selected stimuli (cues) in the environment. The stimulus has to be encoded and recognized '. . . associated correctly with a category (or person). This is a high level process that requires learning and remembering' (Atkinson 1993).

Coded memories of patterns are stored in various ways as mental representations. Opinions vary as to how this is achieved; some theorists propose that information is stored in long-term memory in the form of visual or verbal representations, whereas the propositional theory of coding states that it is abstract and concerned with meanings. There is research evidence to support both theories.

The therapist uses pattern recognition continually in order to identify medical conditions, or familiar problem situations or patterns of dysfunction. Patterns must be matched to those stored in memory. The memory store is searched using top-down and bottom-up strategies which enable recognition to occur. The memory is able to 'flash up' a potential match very quickly when the pattern is familiar. Pattern recognition is used during the generation of hypotheses.

So, for example, if the OT sees a patient sitting slumped in a chair, weeping, reluctant to talk or participate in activity, she may identify a potential pattern of depression. The cues acquired include posture, sad expression, lack of verbalization, and lack of purposeful activity. The therapist can generate a hypothesis about the nature of the problem — 'this patient may be depressed'. However, the wise therapist will not jump from a hypothesis — an explanation which needs testing — to an assumption — a statement accepted as true for the purposes of action. The hypothesis must first be tested.

In this example the therapist might talk to the patient to see if depressive thoughts are expressed; she may talk to other staff to see what their impressions are, and she will look in the patient's case history to see if there is a diagnosis of depression.

If the pattern match continues, the therapist may decide to proceed on the assumption that the patient is depressed. But the pattern may not match; the patient may be recently bereaved, but not clinically depressed; the emotional lability, slumped posture and lack of speech could be due to a stroke or a head injury, the lack of engagement in activity to inappropriate environment or lack of meaningful opportunities for engagement. All these (and more) might be in the therapist's mind as alternative hypotheses to be tested.

Information contributing to pattern recognition may be stored in various forms: as a prototype or stereotype — a typical example of a person or object; as a schema — abstract representation of events, objects and relationships in the real world; as a frame — a data structure representing a stereotypic situation; as cognitive maps; or as templates, which enable the whole pattern to be matched at once.

Experts can develop a store of many thousands of patterns as 'chunks' in which both the pattern and the action it requires are stored together and appropriate responses appear rapidly as soon as the pattern is detected.

Productions, scripts and procedures

The cognitive aspects of problem solving have been described in Chapter 2. Actions or cognitive strategies required to solve problems may be stored as procedures (sequences of actions) which can be encoded as production systems or 'mini-procedures'. Productions link to form sets which together form the behaviour for a larger task. A production may be stored as a simple formula 'if X happens, then do Y', possibly modified by some other circumstance, 'provided that . . .'.

Actions may also be stored in the form of a script, a stereotypic sequence of actions appropriate to a situation — once the situation is identified the actions can be smoothly sequenced according to the script. An example of a script which is often given is that of a child's birthday party — you know at once that party food will include cakes and ice-cream or jelly, that there will be a birthday cake with candles, people will give presents, sing 'Happy Birthday', and the children will play games (or whatever pattern of celebration is culturally appropriate).

There is some evidence that therapists acquire scripts for some of their familiar actions and situations, for example a script for a first interview or a particular form of assessment (Hagedorn 1995b).

Can one learn how to reason more effectively?

It might seem that the answer ought to be 'yes' — that if you understand more about how your mind and memory operate, and about the uses of logic, the laws of probability and formal analytical information processing techniques, you should become a more effective reasoner. An understanding of cognitive psychology, especially in relation to information processing, is certainly useful.

Unfortunately, the evidence from studies of structured attempts to teach medical students more effective forms of reasoning, or better problem solving, have not been very conclusive. In general, such training makes less difference than one might expect, although the more closely it is linked to actual practice — for example realistic role-plays and simulations of real problems or patients — the better.

It may be that there is simply no substitute for rich and varied experience in real clinical situations. However, there is some evidence that considering such experience in an active, critical and reflective manner does help to develop good reasoning skills over a period of time.

DEVELOPING A PERSONAL MODEL

Each therapist is an individual with a unique experience of life both personal and professional. You have your own personal world, your own meanings and associations. Even if you went to the same training college as someone else you cannot guarantee that your experiences there, or what you remember, will be the same as the other person's. As you practice as a therapist you will build on your basic training in an individual way. Whilst OT *is* recognizably OT in most countries, if you speak to any ten individual therapists you are likely to get ten different versions of OT.

It has, therefore, been suggested that each therapist develops what is in effect a personal version of OT — a 'personal model' (or paradigm) (Kortman 1994; Tornebohm 1991).

Having reviewed the personal nature of clinical reasoning it becomes easy to see how this happens. The occupational therapist has her own set of values attitudes and opinions about OT theory (a personal version of the paradigm). The stored memories of lectures, courses, books and papers, the solutions, productions, scripts and procedures, and the images of past patients will all contribute to this personal model.

At one level this is exciting and challenging; many of the applied frames of reference and OT models presented in this book probably originated from the personal model of the author. OT needs the impetus of personal model building in order to develop its theory and practice. It needs therapists who can capture, analyse and communicate their personal practice for the benefit of others.

At another level there needs to be a note of caution. The therapist does need to review her personal model at intervals to check that it has not deviated from currently accepted practice or become stale or out of date. That new idea, that exciting technique may be very good and very interesting — *but is it OT?* A personal model may pick up unconnected material, and needs periodic 'spring-cleaning'. One must return to descriptions of the OT paradigm, and use these to check one's personal version for consistency.

The practitioner must also guard against becoming over-automated, a situation particularly likely to occur when treating very familiar types of cases where reasoning is so smoothed out and habitual that 'the formula' is used as a substitute for original thought.

Reflecting on personal practice and discussing

it with others, using supervision actively, and keeping up to date with the professional literature are important ways of keeping 'on track'.

Reflective practice

There are many techniques which aid reflective practice: keeping a personal diary of ideas, feelings and experiences; discussing cases with others; telling therapeutic 'stories' and learning from them. It is also useful to try more structured analytical techniques, for example trying to recapture all the elements of a situation, to relive it to see what the 'hidden agenda' might have been, and then to alter the 'script', to rehearse different actions and reactions, testing them against what actually happened.

However it is achieved, it is the quality, depth and efficacy of clinical reasoning which differentiates the novice from the competent practitioner, and the competent practioner from the expert (Benner 1984; Slater & Cohn 1991).

Conceptual foundations for practice

6

Primary frames of reference

As described in Chapter 4, there are two types of frames of reference: *primary*, which contains 'borrowed knowledge' derived from sources external to OT (concept 2), and *applied*, a synthesis and interpretation of that knowledge for use in OT which I have called 'the OT version' (concept 3). To avoid repetition I will use the abbreviation PFR to indicate primary frames of reference and AFR to indicate applied ones. (The distinction is useful but academic: in practice if may be simplest to use 'frame of reference' as an umbrella term.)

A primary frame of reference contains theories and knowledge which have been evolved within one of the basic sciences. When knowledge is complex it may be divided into branches, or described according to a particular perspective or set of theories. Primary frames of reference which are relevant to occupational therapy are those which contain information about how a human being functions in her daily life and propose explanations to account for dysfunction.

Occupational therapy has been informed by theories from many different primary frames of reference (see list on page 33). However, these have not all resulted in applied frames of reference. In some cases, just one or two ideas have filtered into OT, whilst in other cases a whole set of theory and practice has been adopted and adapted. Two important primary frames of reference which have resulted in 'OT versions' are:

- the physiological frame of reference
- the psychological frame of reference.

Because occupational therapists deal with human performance, during which biological and psychological processes must be integrated, they frequently mix elements from primary frames of reference when formulating an applied frame of reference. For an AFR to be effective, however, this synthesis must only include compatible elements. It is important, therefore, to remain true to whatever AFR one has selected and to be cautious about using more than one at the same time for the same patient, unless they share a closely related theoretical basis.

THE PHYSIOLOGICAL PRIMARY FRAME OF REFERENCE

The physiological PFR is concerned with the ability of the body to maintain homeostasis in response to internal and external changes. Electrochemical processes control actions, reactions and the individual's ability to respond to and learn from the environment. Performance depends on genetic potential and the integrity and interactions of all body systems, principally the musculoskeletal system, cardiovascular system, neurological system, endocrine system and the special senses.

The internal mechanisms of homeostasis are of background interest to the therapist, but not the main concern. In order to maintain homeostasis the individual must drink, eat, avoid danger, move around in the environment, keep sufficiently warm and so forth. Whilst these actions are partly controlled by automatic bodily processes, they also require active participation by the individual to ensure that the necessities of survival are obtained. The person needs to:

- move and perform functional actions within the environment
- perceive, interpret, and react adaptively to, environmental stimuli.

It is these aspects which concern the therapist. Thus, this PFR has given rise to various applied frames of reference (AFR) (with associated approaches) of which the following are the most important:

- the biomechanical AFR (concerned with functional movement)
- the neurodevelopmental AFR (concerned with development or re-education of motor control)
- the cognitive perceptual AFR (concerned with the way we perceive and interpret our surroundings).

In order to understand the basis of functional movement, occupational therapists need a good foundation knowledge of human anatomy, physiology, and kinesiology, and a detailed understanding of neurophysiology and development.

THE PSYCHOLOGICAL PRIMARY FRAME OF REFERENCE

Psychology deals with the scientific study of behaviour and mental processes. As psychology has evolved during the current century various theories have become influential in their turn.

Psychology began by being closely linked to neurophysiology, then moved into studying behaviour, human development, psychological aspects of learning, and cognition. The development of personal identity and personality and the behaviour of people in groups has also been studied.

Atkinson (1993) describes distinct psychological perspectives:

- biological (the neurobiological basis of behaviour and perception)
- behavioural (learnt responses to environmental stimuli)
- cognitive (study of mental processes of reasoning and learning)
- psychoanalytic (study of unconscious processes)
- phenomenological (concerned with subjective inner experiences).

Psychology has given birth to a variety of specialities—for example, experimental, educational, industrial, environmental, evolutionary, cognitive, social, and clinical.

All the schools of psychology have been influential in occupational therapy in different ways at different times. It has to be admitted that,

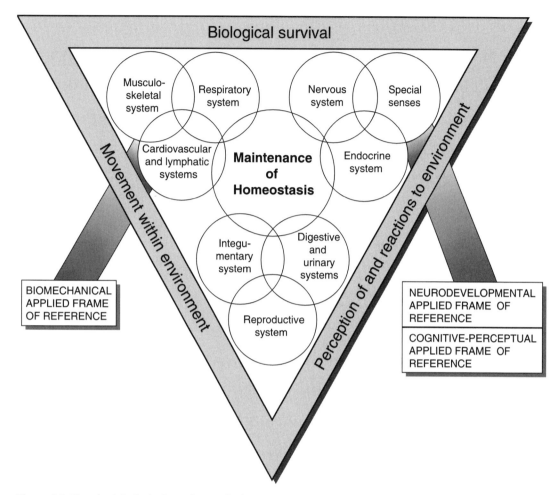

Figure 6.1 The physiological primary frame of reference.

like education (or, indeed, OT itself), psychology is prone to 'fashions' as each new and attractive theory is proposed and gains supporters.

During the 1980s, cognitive psychology, which deals with cognitive processes such as memory, information processing and problem solving, has been influential. Social psychology, defined as 'the scientific field that seeks to understand the nature and causes of human behaviour in social situations' (Baron & Byrne 1987), has also been very influential.

An understanding of a range of psychological theories is essential if the therapist is to assess and identify the individual's difficulties in perception, memory, learning and performance, and therefore to construct more effective ways of presenting information or improving skills. It is also important to understand the influence of culture, and other people, and to appreciate that each person creates a personal world of meanings, symbols and memories.

Psychological perspectives and applied frames of reference

The biological basis of behaviour

The biological perspective overlaps with the physiological PFR since it deals with how the brain receives and interprets information from sensory receptors and integrates this with behaviour. This has been incorporated into the spatiotemporal and sensory integration approaches and also the cognitive perceptual AFR (concerned with the identification and treatment of perceptual deficits, usually following brain damage).

Behaviourism

Behaviourism is primarily a theory of learning. This has developed from the original research into stimulus response learning by Pavlov, Thorndike and Watson, followed by the work on operant conditioning by Skinner and many others. Research is concentrated on proposing explanations of observable human behaviour in terms of interaction with the environment. The environment provides stimuli to which the individual responds. The individual is able to appreciate the outcome of the response by means of feedback. Responses which are rewarded or are useful to the individual in satisfying drives are continued and become part of the behavioural repertoire. Those which are unsuccessful, or which achieve unpleasant results, are discontinued.

'Hard line' behaviourists believe that the individual has little choice in deciding how to behave, being 'programmed' to react through conditioning derived from past experience. All interior motivators such as emotions and thoughts as discounted either as products of behaviour, or as internal, unobservable, and therefore incapable of objective study.

Bandura extended the concept of operant conditioning and recognized that the individual does not need to experience the reinforcement personally, but may learn by observing the results of the behaviour of others, a process called *modelling* which has important implications for therapy.

Other researchers have moved away from the extreme behaviourist position and have tended to include some elements of cognitive theory, particularly aspects of the information processing theories of memory, learning and decision making.

Few occupational therapists apply the behavioural frame of reference in strict and unadapted form, but behavioural theories have been influential in both education and therapy, and are used in behavioural modification and desensitization programmes, and in skill training and programmed learning.

A feature of all such programmes is the breaking down of tasks into simple component parts and sequences and the use of very clear statements of objectives, goals and methods of instruction, and of schedules of reinforcement, designed to meet the learning needs of the individual.

Behaviourism had led to the behavioural AFR (training skills by a process of behavioural modification) and has been adapted and extended by the inclusion of cognitive psychology to form the cognitive-behavioural AFR (dealing with the links between thoughts, feelings and actions).

Cognitive psychology

Cognitive psychologists, in direct contrast to the behaviourists, are primarily concerned with understanding the processes of the mind such as perception, memory and conceptualization and to provide theories about how the individual forms relationships between concepts, interprets structures and makes sense of the environment. Since these processes cannot, like behaviours, be directly observed, much has to be done by inference and by constructing models to explain various mental processes. Links are made between the effectiveness with which the individual manages these processes, and her ability to learn and develop rules, skills, and roles, and to plan and carry out appropriate behaviour.

Different theories have evolved combining the physiology of cognition, elements of learning theory or elements of developmental or humanistic theories in various proportions.

Early cognitive research was aimed at discovering the nature of intelligence, and whether this could be influenced in any way, but this form of research has largely been superceded. More recently, researchers have used sophisticated technology to investigate the physiological changes which occur in the brain as a result of perceiving or learning, and have attempted to identify which parts of the brain are responsible for specific cognitive functions. Despite this research, a great deal is still unknown about the nature of thought and the means whereby information is actually stored and processed.

Other cognitive psychologists seek to use their theories and models of mental processes to enable them to predict how an individual is likely to behave in a given situation. They see the ability of the individual to learn insightfully, to solve problems, to use his past experiences and to plan his future actions as important. The individual's internal constructs of past, present, and particularly the future, are of significance. The work of Bruner (a cognitive psychologist/educational theorist) has influenced the models of some American OT theorists, especially his work on meaning as a component of human learning and behaviour (Bruner 1990). Bandura moved away from strict behaviourism and proposed that perceptions of self-efficacy (self-confidence in the performance of activities) was important [Bandura 1977a]).

Information processing theories have been used to model the process of learning and remembering and a new discipline of cognitive science has evolved to link this work with that on artificial intelligence.

Cognitive approaches to the treatment of psychiatric illness or personality disorder have been developed. These approaches tend to emphasize the link between faulty ways of thinking and feeling or of perceiving the world, with various mental disorders, especially those associated with anxiety, depression and stress.

For example, Ellis introduced *rational emotive therapy*, summarized by the ABC theory: **A**— Antecedent, a fact, event, behaviour or attitude which **B** influences the patient's **B**elief which **C** decides the **C**onsequence. He also coined the expression 'musterbatory behaviour' to describe acts originating from irrational compulsive belief patterns.

Beck developed *cognitive therapy*, a less directive and interpretive style, based on helping the client to analyse the interactions of his thoughts,

emotions and behaviours. Other workers look for 'life themes' persistent rules or attitudes which predominate in and direct the client's behaviour.

Cognitive-behavioural approaches are structured, and rely on methods which seek to change the content of thought, particularly anxious, depressive or obsessive thought patterns, thereby improving affect and behaviour.

Other approaches incorporate the theory of social modelling, or techniques of behavioural rehearsal or role-play. Techniques such as reality orientation and reminiscence therapy are also cognitive in origin, since they link the individual's perceptions and memories to current events.

The cognitive perspective has led to the development of the cognitive-perceptual AFR, the cognitive-behavioural AFR, and the cognitive disabilities model (Allen; linking levels of skill to levels of cognitive development; see Chapter 10). (Cognitive-analytical approaches and brief-focused cognitive analytical therapy have also been developed but these are not mentioned widely in OT texts.)

Psychoanalysis

The psychoanalytic or *psychodynamic* perspective is derived partly from the study of the disorders of mental processes which are seen in psychiatry and partly from theories proposed by various psychologists, psychoanalysts and psychotherapists. The term 'psychodynamic' has been used as an umbrella term (rather than the more restrictive 'analytic') to include the different, but related, theories which are concerned with the origins of an individual's personality and motivation, and with methods of helping the individual to gain insight, to achieve personal growth and to meet personal needs.

The psychodynamic perspective is unique in dealing with the unconscious motivations for actions, interations and beliefs, and/or the symbolic content of images and perceptions. Explanations for the unconscious basis of behaviour differ, and include psychoanalytical theory, object relations theory, psychotherapy theories, and some elements of cognitive and developmental psychology and learning theory. This is an area where theorists abound and generalizations are difficult: two distinct applied frames of reference will be described:

- the analytical AFR (derived from psychoanalytical and object relations theories)
- the group work AFR (derived from group theory and psychotherapy).

Social psychology

Social psychology has contributed to our understanding of people as they form opinions of others, make relationships and operate in groups, and of the effects of culture and society. It deals with attitudes, motivation and the behavioural expression of emotions such as aggression. Social psychology has not resulted directly in an AFR, but has been incorporated into the group work AFR, and has influenced other AFR and OT Models.

Humanistic psychology

Humanistic psychology needs to be distinguished from 'humanism' which is a philosophy concerned with the nature of humanity, personal consciousness and individual being. Humanism influenced the development of humanistic psychology and humanistic educational theory. Humanism takes a strongly atheistic standpoint, however, humanistic psychology does not preclude religious belief.

Humanistic psychology is described as phenomenological because it is concerned with subjective individual experience, the personal 'world view' that each individual develops as a result of his unique life, feelings and perceptions.

Influential theorists are Maslow (self-actualization), Frankl (personal meaning), Kelly (personal construct) and Rogers (person centred counselling and person centred learning).

These theorists emphasize the essentially positive nature of every individual, who should be valued and will respond accordingly. The individual has the potential to control her life and to choose what she wishes to become. She can only

change and progress if she wills to do so; change can only take place if it is an active process which is meaningful to the individual. Positive change can occur throughout life. Living should be a celebratory, joyful experience.

Important concepts in the humanistic view of personal relationships are the need for authenticity—being one's true self—honesty, and non-judgemental regard and respect for others. These theories have become very influential in psychotherapy, teaching, social work and OT, and linked with some developmental and cognitive theories. There are many natural resonances between person centred theories and the fundamental philosophy of occupational therapy as expressed by its American founders (long before humanistic psychology had been developed).

Carl Rogers has been very significant in the move from teacher/therapist centred, directive approaches to student/client centred ones. He felt that therapists should act as counsellors or facilitators, providing resources and enabling people to learn and change. He saw learning as a life-long search for individual meaning, fulfilment, growth and self-knowledge. His ideas were based on personal experience as a teacher and counsellor, backed up by the anecdotal accounts of others.

Key features of Rogerian counselling or psychotherapy are that it is person centred, uses a non-directive style, avoids interpretation, reflects back to the individual her ideas, perceptions and beliefs and provides encouragement for her to search for personal meaning and self-actualization. Humanists believe that it is theoretically possible, by means of counselling, for an individual to achieve a large degree of self-knowledge and control over her own life.

The humanistic perspective has been criticized for promoting unrealistic starry-eyed optimism and, whilst the ideals are given lip-service by many, they are frequently not put into practice, not least because many of the systems within which health care is delivered make it difficult to allow the amount of time and the degree of freedom of coice for the client which is required. In reality, the opportunity for the individual to control, direct and shape her own life may be minimal and, whilst choice may be beneficial, some

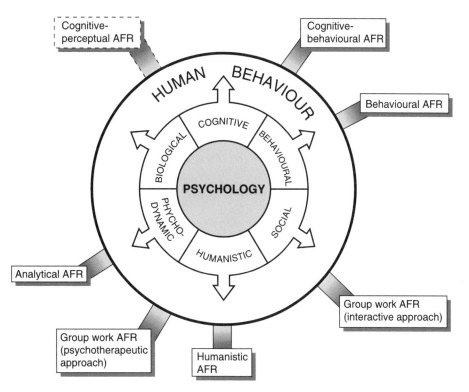

Figure 6.2 The psychological primary frame of reference.

clients are overwhelmed by being presented with too much of it.

The amount of expertise and training required to use humanistic techniques such as client centred counselling is also frequently underestimated: whilst basic counselling skills can be acquired quite readily by most therapists, it should be recognized that clients requiring long-term or in-depth counselling should be referred to a suitably qualified counsellor or psychotherapist.

A number of holistic, humanistic psychotherapies have evolved, frequently combining elements of cognitive or developmental theories with humanism and psychotherapy, including:

- gestalt therapy (Perls)
- rational emotive therapy (Ellis)
- personal construct (repertory grid) (Kelly; Bannister & Fransella)
- transactional analysis (Berne)
- psychosynthesis (Assagioli)
- person centred counselling (Maslow; Rogers)

Box 6.1   Summary of applied frames of reference and approaches

Applied frames of reference	Approach
Biomechanical	Graded activities Activities of daily living Compensatory
Neurodevelopmental	Bobath PNF Rood Conductive education Sensory integration Spatiotemporal Sensory stimulation
Behavioural	Behavioural modification
Cognitive-behavioural	Cognitive-behavioural
Cognitive-perceptual	Cognitive-perceptual
Analytical	Freudian/neo-Freudian Object relations
Group work	Psychotherapeutic Interactive/activities
Humanistic	Person centred Student centred

- encounter groups (Rogers)
- co-counselling (Jackins)
- theme centred group work (Cohn).

In the context of OT, the humanistic AFR has produced two approaches, the person centred approach (incorporating various person centred counselling techniques) and the student centred approach (based largely on Rogerian principles of education).

Applied frames of reference and approaches

Each AFR can be put into practice by means of one or more approaches. These are sets of compatible assessments, forms of intervention, treatment techniques and styles of therapeutic relationship by means of which theories are translated into action. These are described in Chapters 7 and 8.

7

Applied frames of reference which focus on physical dysfunction

THE BIOMECHANICAL APPLIED FRAME OF REFERENCE

The biomechanical AFR is used almost exclusively in the context of the process of physical rehabilitation. The connection is so close that the two are often confused, but the rehabilitation process is a much larger entity than the biomechanical AFR, which is just one of the AFRs which can be used to provide a framework for rehabilitation.

The 'bio' part of the title is based on kinesiology, which combines neuromuscular physiology, musculoskeletal anatomy and biomechanics. The 'mechanics' part indicates that it is also based on 'mechanical' laws, e.g. leverage, gravity, friction, and resistance. In this AFR the therapist focuses on 'the body as a machine', usually working to improve one or more of 'the four Ss'—suppleness, strength, stability and stamina—and through this to improve function. Physical exercise, isotonic or isometric, is used to increase the strength and bulk of muscles and to improve stamina and work tolerance. Repetitive exercise is also used to increase or restore the range of movement at a joint.

To improve function one needs to practice and to work at the upper edge of current abilities. In a typical training or retraining programme the individual is required to work as close to his functional limits as possible, without undue fatigue, and the 'goal posts' are continually moved as improvement occurs. Grading of the elements in the exercise programme, e.g. adding assistance or resistance, altering range, speed, duration and repetition, is often a crucial part of the therapist's role.

The biomechanical AFR has several approaches which may be used separately or at different stages in the treatment programme. Those commonly described include: the graded activities approach, the activities of daily living (ADL) approach, and the compensatory approach.

The graded activities approach uses activities for remedial purposes, not necessarily because the person wants or needs to engage in them in his daily life. Activities may include craft techniques, 'DIY', sports, games and so forth. Many accounts of the biomechanical AFR are limited to this approach, transferring the others I have listed to 'rehabilitation'.

In this approach the performance of an activity is used to produce specific effects, for example to promote defined movements, to exercise specific muscle groups, or to work for extended tolerance of standing, sitting or walking.

Thorough physical assessment and measurement of function is an essential precursor to therapy. Precise measurements must be made to set a baseline from which subsequent improvement can be assessed. Measurements can include: joint range (using a goniometer), muscle power, length of time a movement or activity can be sustained, speed, number of repetitions, distance, or any other precisely quantifiable factor. The selected factor must be reassessed at regular intervals in order to monitor progress and set new targets.

In order for this approach to be effective, elements in the performance must be controlled and graded with precision. This requires an imaginative and ingenious attitude on the part of the therapist, which in former times led to the use of complex adaptive apparatus, pulley circuits and the like. The use of productive activities in this way involves thought and preparation, and unless correctly used and monitored, the activity may be too generalized in effect to be useful.

It is almost inevitable that patient choice in the selection of an activity will be limited by the constraints of meeting specific physical objectives, and the product must often be subordinated to the process. This approach has been criticized as overly directive and mechanistic; it has also, ironically, been criticized as insufficiently precise. This, together with the reaction against 'craft work' and the desire to appear technologically advanced, has resulted in the use of stereotyped non-productive activities (such as remedial 'games') purely for their exercise value, and not for any intrinsic interest or end product. This trend was very noticeable during the mid 1970s, but it is now decreasing.

There is currently a renewed interest in the specific remedial use of activities as it is once more appreciated that the combined psychological and physical benefits of constructive, practical or creative activities may outweigh the disadvantages of any lack of precision in physical application.

Some interesting adaptations to computers have recently been produced, together with equipment using surface electrodes to translate specific muscle contraction into switching of electric apparatus. This is sometimes used in connection with biofeedback techniques.

The accelerated pace of recovery from trauma due to improved medical and surgical techniques during the past two decades has rendered rehabilitation unnecessary in some cases and has generally resulted in much shorter hospitalization, which has left little time for graded activity programmes to be implemented. The graded activities approach is therefore mainly used to treat individuals with more serious injuries or conditions requiring longer-term treatment, which is often undertaken on an out-patient basis.

There are some individuals who just cannot relate to this approach; it is my personal view that patients whose needs are better met by exercise than activity, or who actually prefer exercises, should be referred to a physiotherapist.

The activities of daily living (ADL) approach is concerned with the movement components of functional activity. It uses biomechanical principles to improve the individual's ability to do personal or domestic activities of daily living. A basic assumption of this approach is 'practice makes perfect'—that by repeated practice, by continually challenging the individual to do a little more, praising achievements and consolidating gains by continued use of the regained skill, function will improve.

> **Q** Where do you stand on the question of the use of activities for specific physical treatment? How far should activities be adapted? Is adaptation effective? Is it too time-consuming? Should OT's use non-productive 'activities'? How do patients react to this form of therapy? Discuss these points with some colleagues: you may well get a wide range of firmly held opinions.

The compensatory approach is concerned with enabling people to make up for residual disability by the use of orthoses, prostheses, aids to daily living or home adaptations. This approach may come in quite early in an intervention, when the patient's abilities are limited and aids are therefore necessary. In this situation it may be possible to phase out the use of aids as recovery takes place. Alternatively, the compensatory approach may follow on from the ADL approach or graded activities approach, solving residual problems as the patient prepares to return home or go back to work.

This approach may also involve training in new skills, and requires a good deal of planning, problem solving and lateral thinking on behalf of both patient and therapist. The approach may be quite mechanistic, merely looking at assistive devices, but in a more adaptive form other compensatory changes may be needed, involving attitudinal changes and adoption of techniques such as time management, energy conservation, joint protection, pacing of activities, and lifestyle planning.

In the community the compensatory approach is much used, since getting the home environment right for a disabled individual can make a major contribution to personal independence.

Summary of the biomechanical applied frame of reference

Metamodel: Reductionist.
Origin of problem: An illness, injury or congenital disorder has affected the strength, range or coordination of bodily movement, with consequent limitation of normal function for the individual.

Primary assumptions
- The application of a graded programme of exercise based on kinesiological principles will restore normal or near normal function.
- Biomechanical principles can be used to provide aids, orthoses or adaptive equipment to overcome residual disability.
- 'Practice makes perfect'.

Terminology: Patient; therapist; disability; function.
Patient/therapist relationship: The therapist prescribes, directs and advises, the patient actively cooperates.
Examples of applications: Hand injuries; fractures, peripheral nerve lesions, amputees; burns; cardiac conditions.
Approaches: Graded activities; activities of daily living; compensatory.

Examples of techniques
- Graded activities approach
  - graded physical treatment: e.g. to promote muscle power, joint range, endurance
  - adapted activities: craft and technical
  - adapted apparatus: e.g. cycles, lathes, pulleys, springs, special handles
  - remedial games—using adapted equipment
  - some forms of biofeedback
- ADL approach
  - ADL practice to promote range, strength and stamina and effective functional performance
- Compensatory approach
  - adapted equipment for activities of daily living
  - home adaptations
  - assessment for and provision of wheelchairs and adapted vehicles
  - provision of, and training in use of orthoses, prostheses.

Criteria for evaluation of outcome: The patient will show measurable improvement in physical function.

Advantages: Biomechanical techniques are well researched and can be shown to produce improvement in physical function. Because improving functional ability is the chief goal and results are relatively rapid, the patient can see positive benefits as treatment progresses and is motivated to continue. Residual disabilities can be overcome by aids and orthoses.

Disadvantages: Because treatment in the graded activities approach has to be very specific to produce results, patient choice in the selection of activities may be restricted: there is a danger that programmes may become stereotyped. Activity programmes take time to set up and prepare and are impractical where treatment time is limited. An overly physical bias may result in wider social, environmental or psychological problems being ignored.

SUGGESTED READING

The references given below are quite specific, but you will also find relevant material in the references quoted for the rehabilitation model.

Galley P M, Forster A L 1987 Human Movement, 2nd edn. Churchill Livingstone, Edinburgh. *Basic review of anatomy, movement mechanics and principles of exercise (for physiotherapy students).*

Kielhofner G 1992 Conceptual foundations of occupational therapy. F A Davis, Philadelphia

Mills D, Fraser C 1989 Therapeutic activities for the upper limb. Winslow Press, Bicester. *Ch. 6: The biomechanical model.*

Norkin C, White J 1985 Measurement of joint motion. F A Davis

Pedretti L (ed) Occupational Therapy: practice skills for physical dysfunction, 2nd edn. C V Mosby. *Chs 5, 6, 7, 8, 9, 18.*

Trombley C A 1989 Occupational therapy for physical dysfunction, 3rd edn. Williams & Wilkins. Part Three: Biomechanical approach. Part Five: Rehabilitative approach.

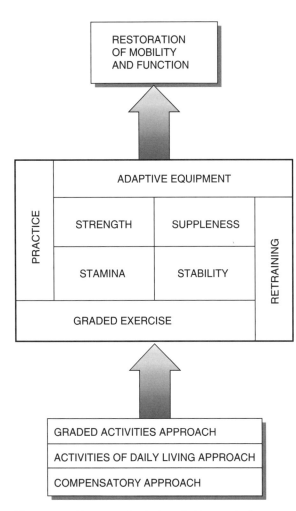

Figure 7.1 The biomechanical applied frame of reference.

THE NEURODEVELOPMENTAL APPLIED FRAME OF REFERENCE

The neurodevelopmental AFR is based on principles of motor control, neuromuscular facilitation and sensory integration and has a strongly developmental base. Various techniques and approaches have been evolved for use in the treatment of physical disorders, psychiatric disorders, paediatric disorders and learning disabilities (mental handicap).

In several cases the primary techniques associated with an approach were evolved by physiotherapists, do not involve functional patterns of movement, and, in unadapted form, are not readily related to activity based occupational therapy, being more commonly used as an adjunct to or precursor of it. However, it is possible, for example, to adapt Bobath positioning for use in functional activity, and to incorporate basic neurodevelopmental principles into an activity based OT programme.

In general, the emphasis is on the sequence of interventions and the use of sensory and perceptual input and voluntary or reflex output to promote the attainment of, and progression through, stages of increasing skill and complexity to a point where potential has been developed to the maximum possible for the individual.

The approaches associated with this AFR are referred to in some texts as models or frames of reference in their own right (see suggested reading). When used by a very experienced therapist who has specialized in a field, e.g. paediatrics, the depth of knowledge and expertise being used may well justify this. However, far more often these techniques are used at a less expert level by therapists who also use other approaches in their work, and I feel that 'approach' is therefore a more logical classification in this introductory text.

The fact that techniques originating in these approaches are sometimes used at a rather low level of skill leads me to sound a note caution. In general, neurodevelopmental techniques require considerable practice and skill and should not be employed by people who do not really understand what they are doing. It is not necessary to be an expert, but it is necessary to be competent, as incorrect use is at best ineffective, and at worst damaging.

Approaches include:

- Bobath approach
- PNF (proprioceptive neuromuscular facilitation) approach
- Conductive education
- Rood approach
- Sensory integration
- Spatiotemporal adaptation
- Sensory stimulation.

Approaches

Bobath approach (syn. motor control)

A bilateral approach to the treatment of hemiplegia or spasticity utilizing positioning, weightbearing, reflex inhibition and sensory facilitation. This can be adapted for use with OT activities more readily than some other techniques (Bobath 1986) and is widely used by occupational therapists.

Basic principles include:

- Positioning the patient in a manner which will inhibit the development of abnormal reflexes and synergies and reduce abnormal muscle tone enabling the patient to relearn normal movement patterns.
- Facilitating correct movement by positioning, correct handling, use of sensory stimulation and the use of key control points on the body.
- Working through a developmental sequence — lying, 'all-fours', trunk control, sitting, standing, weight transfer, stepping, walking.
- Involving both sides of the body in all activities. Use of activities which *promote*: crossing the midline with the arm; diagonal patterns of arm use; special bilateral grip; weightbearing through affected side; trunk rotation; and which *avoid*: flexor patterns in the upper limb and extensor patterns in the lower limb; stimulation of associated reactions.

PNF approach

The technique uses positioning and diagonal patterns of movement in developmental sequence and emphasizes sensory input, visual cues and verbal commands to produce maximum input. Sensory input stimulates and facilitates motor output. This approach is less adaptable for use in OT, except as an adjunct to therapy, but some general principles are transferable.

Conductive education approach (Peto)

A highly structured and formal system mainly used with children (although some work has been done with adults), based on a planned, intensive, programme aimed at achieving goals for each individual following a blend of cognitive and neurodevelopmental principles. The therapist acts as a 'conductor' planning tasks, facilitating movement, and using formalized verbalization to assist actions—the patient also says what he is doing at each stage as he does it. Personal control and responsibility are emphasized; rhythm is used to promote and initiate movement. Conductive education is currently attracting considerable interest and is used by physiotherapists, but it is not as yet widely used by British occupational therapists. It requires special training. Some therapists have incorporated the concept of patient verbalization as an adjunct to other therapy.

Rood approach

This uses similar principles to sensory integration and PNF but emphasizes tactile stimulation (brushing; icing; tapping; pressure, and stretch reflexes). Rood is both an OT and a physiotherapist but the technique is more related to PT than OT. Occupational therapists tend to use it as a precursor to other therapy.

Sensory integration approach (Ayres) (King)

In the treatment of children with developmental difficulties, and children or adults with psychiatric disorders or mental handicap, the emphasis is on the capacity of the individual to perceive and react correctly to people and the environment. Recognizing the strong link between sensory input and motor output, the therapist may use sensorimotor activity to stimulate perception and proprioception, thus raising the general level of activity where this is retarded.

In this approach development is depicted as a spiral in which the individual gradually moves upwards, having consolidated gains at each level. The importance of the integration and interpretation of all sensory inputs, and the necessity of promoting integrated sensory stimulation to develop or restore function, are stressed. The link between sensory input, cortical organization, and personal appreciation of the use of adaptive skills is important.

Activity (such as play) using touch, vibration, sound, smell, colour, is geared to stimulation at subcortical level, with particular attention to vestibular and proprioceptive input. This technique was developed by Ayres for use with children and neurologically damaged adults.

Another version of the technique has been used in a psychiatric setting following the work by King with schizophrenics; she advocated the use of activities which increase and promote vestibular stimulation, bilateral integration and the integration of primitive postural reflexes to overcome synaptic barriers and promote normal body image, posture, righting reactions and reflexes.

Both approaches are complex and require considerable study, so it is essential to read the longer descriptions given in the reading list.

Spatiotemporal adaptation approach

This is similar in some ways to the sensory integration approach. It is also designed for use with children. One of its main assumptions is that interaction with the environment shapes development, which is again seen as a spiral process. Occupation is seen as a context which provides purpose and motivation which help to promote and shape motor performance. Again, this is a complex approach which requires careful study and practice.

Sensory stimulation

This approach is used to provide richly stimulating input to one or more senses. To achieve this, colour, scents, sound, texture, movement, vibration, flashing lights, and different types of touch are used to promote a reaction. The quality of the reaction will depend on whether the combination of sensory inputs produces a relaxation response or stimulates alertness and attention. This approach is most often used with individuals who have a severe learning disability or brain damage. The Snoezelan environment is an example of sensory stimulation.

Summary of the neurodevelopmental AFR

Metamodel: Although many techniques are very precisely directed, developmentally one must regard an individual as an integrated, reactive

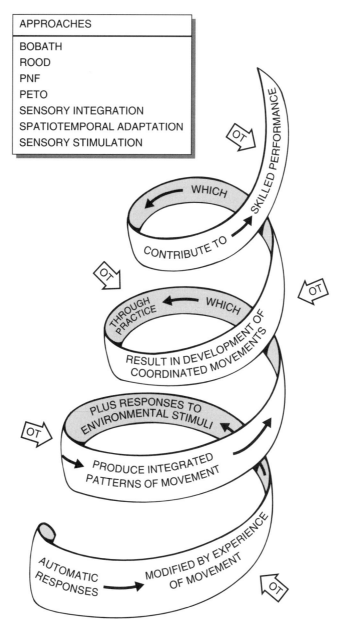

APPROACHES

BOBATH
ROOD
PNF
PETO
SENSORY INTEGRATION
SPATIOTEMPORAL ADAPTATION
SENSORY STIMULATION

Figure 7.2 The neurodevelopmental applied frame of reference.

person in whom a deficit in one area will affect the whole. This AFR is therefore organismic in general outlook, although it may become reductionist in application.

Origin of problem: The adult or child shows developmental delay or regression to a primitive neurodevelopmental level due to congenital or acquired damage to the brain, or genetic abnormality or the effects of other illness or injury.

Primary assumptions
● Neurological development occurs in stages:

these stages relate to the acquisition of sensorimotor skills. Stages cannot be 'jumped' or missed. In order to gain or regain function the individual must be taken through a normal developmental sequence.

● There is a strong link between sensory input and motor output.
● Use of proprioception, positioning and reflexes can facilitate normal movement, posture and reactions.

Terminology: Therapist; patient/client; therapy (and the language of the specific neurodevelopmental technique being employed).

Patient/-therapist relationship: The therapist assesses and decides on the intervention, the patient cooperates, actively or passively.

Approaches: Bobath; PNF; Rood; Conductive education; Sensory integration; Spatiotemporal adaptation; Sensory stimulation:

Examples of applications
● Children
  — spasticity; 'clumsy child'; brain damage; mental handicap; dystrophy
● Adults
  — learning difficulties (mental handicap)
  — physical conditions, e.g. cerebral vascular accident, head injury, multiple sclerosis, motor neurone disease, Parkinsonism, spinal cord lesions
  — psychiatric disorders, e.g. schizophrenia, institutionalization, dementia.

Criteria for evaluation of outcome: The individual has achieved improvement in sensorimotor function and/or has achieved the normal patterns of movement responses and abilities for his/her age/sex.

Advantages: When used correctly and intensively these therapies produce good results particularly in preventing the development of abnormal patterns of movement and deformity following neurological damage.

Disadvantages: Unless used intensively, skilfully and correctly by all members of the treatment team, results are likely to be disappointing. Special training is required to use most techniques effectively. Working neurodevelopmentally is time-consuming and functional recovery in the brain damaged adult, e.g. walking, may be delayed with consequent frustration for the patient. The techniques are less suitable for use with very elderly patients. Although vigorously promoted by enthusiasts, there is some recent criticism of the physiological assumptions on which therapy is based; studies are difficult to compare and evaluate and it has been argued that good results are due more to the intensive nature of the treatment, and the excellent rapport which develops between the patient and an expert practitioner, than to the techniques themselves. Extreme, highly intensive, versions of some techniques, particularly as applied to children, are still very controversial.

SUGGESTED READING

Bobath B 1986 Adult hemiplegia: evaluation and treatment, 2nd edn. Heineman, London
Creek J (ed) 1990 Occupational therapy and mental health; principles; skills and practice. Churchill Livingstone, Edinburgh. *Ch. 11: Sensory integration*
Eggers O 1988 Occupational therapy in the rehabilitation of adult hemiplegia. Heineman, London
Finlay L 1988 Occupational therapy practice in psychiatry. Croom Helm, London. *Ch. 2: Ayers.*
Hopkins H, Smith H (eds) 1993 Willard and Spackman's occupational therapy. Williams and Wilkins, Philadelphia. *Ch. 4: Section 3E Neurodevelopmental FR. 3F Sensory integration FR. 3J Spatiotemporal adaptation.*
Kielhofner G 1992 Conceptual foundations of occupational therapy. F A Davis, Philadelphia. *Ch. 11: Motor control model. Ch. 12: Sensory integration model. Ch. 13: Spatiotemporal adaptation.*
Macdonald J 1990 The international course on conductive education at the Peto Andras State Institute for Conductive Education, Budapest. British Journal of Occupational Therapy 53(7): 295–300
Mosey A C 1986 Psychosocial components of occupational therapy. Raven Press. *Ch. 31: Sensory integration.*
Pedretti L (ed) Occupational Therapy: practice skills for physical dysfunction edn. C V Mosby. *Ch. 8: Evaluation of reflexes. Ch. 9: Evaluation of sensation, perception, 2nd cognition. Ch. 13: Neurophysiology of sensorimotor approaches. Ch. 14: Rood. Ch 15: Brunnstrom. Ch. 16: Bobath. Ch. 17: PNF.*
Trombley C A 1989 Occupational therapy for physical dysfunction, 3rd edn. Williams & Wilkins, Baltimore. Part Two: Neurodevelopmental approach.

Zoltan B, Seiv E, Freishtat B 1986 Perceptual and cognitive dysfunction in the adult stroke patient, 2nd edn. Slack, New Jersey

NOTE: these references deal primarily with the application to adults. For use of techniques with children you will need to find specialized literature.

INCOMPATIBLE AFRs

You should by now have realized that the approaches of the biomechanical and neuro-developmental AFRs are incompatible. Although both AFRs are soundly based on physiology, each uses a distinct knowledge base, and the resultant techniques are mutually exclusive.

Unless this is clearly understood there is room for a good deal of confusion and, consequently, ineffective therapy. Practitioners who are old enough to remember the revolution in therapy which occurred during the early 1970s when neurodevelopmental techniques began to take over from biomechanical ones in the treatment of brain damaged patients will recall the frequent and acrimonious arguments between proponents of the opposing views (a debate which has not entirely resolved even now).

As a generalization, the biomechanical AFR is reductionist in philosophy and is used in the rehabilitation of musculoskeletal or peripheral neurological injury, whilst the neurodevelopmental AFR is more holistic and is used in the treatment of trauma or developmental delay/regression affecting the sensorimotor systems in children or adults.

The most significant opposing principles of the two AFRs are summarized in Box 7.1. This does, however, represent a simplification and it must be remembered that application will vary in accordance with the needs of individuals with specific conditions.

THE COGNITIVE-PERCEPTUAL APPLIED FRAME OF REFERENCE

Perception is a cognitive process which involves the interpretation and identification of sensory information within the brain. If damage occurs to the brain, the ability to interpret such information can be affected. This may result in difficulties in performance due to incorrect assumptions

---

Box 7.1 Incompatible AFRs

Neurodevelopmental AFR (Bobath approach)	Biomechanical AFR (graded activities approach)
Work first for control and pattern of gross movements.	Work first for functional use. May promote fine movements.
Always work from proximal to distal.	May work from distal to proximal.
In the upper limb use extensor/abductor patterns. Promote grip last. Avoid stimulation of flexor surfaces.	In the upper limb work for flexion and functional use —promote grip early. May use stimulation of flexor surfaces.
In the lower limb work against extensor thrust and adductor patterns.	In the lower limb promote knee and hip extension and stability of knee and ankle.
Delay walking and standing until developmentally ready.	Stand/walk as early as possible.
Grade therapy according to developmental stages: work within limits of current level until ability to progress is established.	Grade therapy according to progress: work at or just beyond limits of current capacity.
Use orthoses and external supports with discretion and as a last resort.	Use orthoses as routine.
Emphasize treatment of whole body to achieve symmetry.	Emphasize treatment of affected part.
Emphasize sensory integration and proprioception.	Emphasize functional and protective sensation.
Do not encourage compensation by one part of the body for lost function in another.	Encourage compensation for lost function by using a different body part.

about the environment leading to faulty motor control. Knowledge concerning the environment, and also knowledge of patterns of movement which enable appropriate responses to be made when information is received, are also stored in the brain and can be damaged.

The cognitive perceptual AFR is concerned with these 'hidden' mental processes which enable a person to: know where he is; recognize objects or people; move around within a defined space; carry out purposeful movement; learn; remember; use logic; problem solve; cope with use of concrete and abstract language.

Perceptual deficits include many different disorders. Two important groups are the agnosias and the apraxias. It is important to distinguish between a perceptual or cognitive deficit which originates from damage to the parts of the brain which recognize, store and interpret information, and deficits due to damage to the peripheral organs which receive or transmit that information. In agnosias and apraxias there is no physical damage to these organs.

An agnosia (i.e. absence of knowing) is an inability to use information, or recognize a concept which was previously familiar. For example, inability to count objects or to tell the time, inability to recognize a part of one's own body.

An apraxia (i.e. absence of skill) is an inability to perform a previously known skill, although the instruction to do so is understood and the physical ability to do so is intact. This could include getting dressed, manipulating objects, writing or pattern making.

There are other deficits such as visual field problems and body image problems which also cause functional difficulties.

The cognitive perceptual AFR has three approaches: diagnostic, remedial and compensatory.

The diagnostic approach

The *diagnostic approach* requires a very good understanding of neuroanatomy and the complex mechanisms of perception. The therapist uses performance tests and special assessments to identify the type and degree of perceptual deficit. An experienced therapist can often make a diagnosis from observing functional performance just as well as by using tests; deficits in test performance do not always correlate with functional difficulties, but may support a diagnosis.

Having decided what the problem is, the therapist can then decide whether to attempt treatment to improve the ability, or intervention to compensate for the loss. Even if it proves impossible to improve function, it is important to understand the extent of the deficit, which can sometimes be covered by a good social manner or natural adaptability. A perceptual deficit may seriously affect skills such as driving even though motor function is intact.

Perceptual deficits can be hard to diagnose, especially when several are present at once. They may occur in adults with brain damage from a variety of causes who also have other problems which may make diagnosis difficult. Perceptual deficits also occur in children and may be associated with developmental delay, these usually respond to treatment more readily than deficits caused by trauma.

The remedial approach

The *remedial approach* involves training or retraining the perceptual skill by intensive practice, but success in the case of brain damaged adults may be only partial. It is debatable whether improvement is due to the practice, or simply to spontaneous recovery as the acute phase following trauma subsides. One theory which explains recovery deals with 'brain plasticity', i.e. the capacity of the brain to compensate for damage by relearning, and by using unaffected 'spare capacity' to make up for that which has been lost. Another theory deals with the ability to generalize a skill learnt in one context to another, e.g. by practising patterns in order to improve writing, or copying designs in blocks in order to improve spatial awareness. Computers have recently been used to assist in perceptual training.

One of the difficulties in treating severe forms of perceptual deficit is that the patient may be unaware of the problem because the damaged

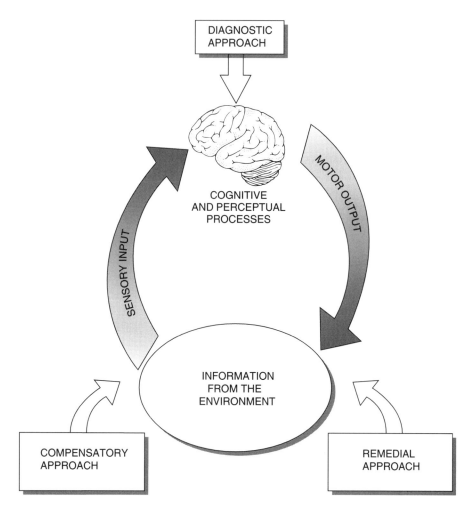

Figure 7.3 The cognitive-perceptual applied frame of reference.

area of the brain has no means of communicating the extent of the damage to the intact areas. There is a gap in a visual field, or a problem in using a part of the body, but the person simply fails to realize the nature and extent of the deficit. It is plainly very difficult to teach someone to compensate for a deficit which, for him, does not exist. It is equally difficult for new learning to occur if perception or memory is affected.

The compensatory approach

The *compensatory approach* involves teaching the individual to use other perceptual abilities, or providing additional cues and prompts in the environment which promote perception. Such cues may include: positioning of objects; breaking down tasks into stages; presentation of information in small quantities; verbal cues; social cues or prompts; use of distinctive colours or shapes to help in identification of objects.

Summary of the cognitive-perceptual AFR

Metamodel: Reductionist: the diagnostic approach is concerned to pin-point the nature of the deficit.

Origin of problem: Damage to the brain; developmental delay/disorder.

Primary assumptions

- Perception and cognition are essential prerequisites for functional performance. If recognition of in-coming information is defective, or an appropriate response cannot be organized, the individual will be unable to perform functional activities.
- It may be possible to improve perceptual or cognitive deficits by intensive practice and retraining.
- It may be possible to assist a person to compensate for perceptual or cognitive deficits.

Terminology: Agnosia; apraxia; praxis; visual field defect; hemianopia; unilateral neglect (and a large number of other technical and medical terms to identify deficits).

Patient/therapist relationship: Therapist takes the lead in identifying the problems and assisting the patient to recover function or compensate for its loss.

Approaches: Diagnostic; Remedial; Compensatory.

Examples of applications: Patients who have suffered brain damage as a result of a head injury, a cerebral vascular event (e.g. stroke), or similar trauma. Developmental disorders in children and adults, 'clumsy child' syndrome.

Criteria for evaluation of outcome: A perceptual or cognitive deficit has been identified; performance has been improved by remedial or compensatory techniques.

Advantages: Deals with an area of function which is frequently ignored by other specialists. Suitable practice or other intervention may improve function.

Disadvantages: The theoretical basis for remediation lacks proof. Tests used are not standardized or well researched, require experience for accurate interpretation and may take time to administer. It may be possible to identify a problem, but not possible to do much to improve the situation. Research is lacking.

SUGGESTED READING

Kielhofner G 1992 Conceptual foundations of occupational therapy. F A Davis, Philadelphia. *Ch. 8: The cognitive-perceptual model.*
Pedretti L (ed) Occupational therapy: practice physical dysfunction, 2nd edn. Mosby, St Louis. Ch. 9: Evaluation of perception and skills for cognition.

Trombly C A 1989 Occupational therapy for physical dysfunction, 3rd edn. Williams and Wilkins, Baltimore. Part Two 7: Cognitive and perceptual evaluation and treatment.
Zoltan B, Seiv E, Frieshtat B 1986 Perceptual and cognitive dysfunction in the adult stroke patient, 2nd edn. Slack, New Jersey.

8

Applied frames of reference which focus on psychosocial dysfunction

THE BEHAVIOURAL APPLIED FRAME OF REFERENCE

The scope and origins of behaviourism have already been described. As its name suggests, the focus of the AFR is on behaviour—observable performance. As an OT technique it is most frequently used with people who have learning disabilities, to teach part skills as a means of building up more complex behaviours, or to remove behaviours which are damaging to the person or others, an approach known as *behaviour modification.* Behavioural principles are also used in psychiatry but, apart from desensitization of phobias or anxiety, it is now more usual to employ a cognitive behavioural approach in this field.

Behaviour modification approach

The techniques of behavioural modification can be used both to teach a desirable behaviour or to remove an undesirable one.

A typical behaviour modification programme might involve:

- Settting a precise behavioural objective for the patient to achieve: this involves detailed task analysis so that a portion of behaviour can be isolated and taught.
- Deciding on a positive reinforcer or reward to be used following successful performance, e.g. food or drink, an enjoyable activity, praise, affection, a privilege. (At this point a behavioural contract specifying both the

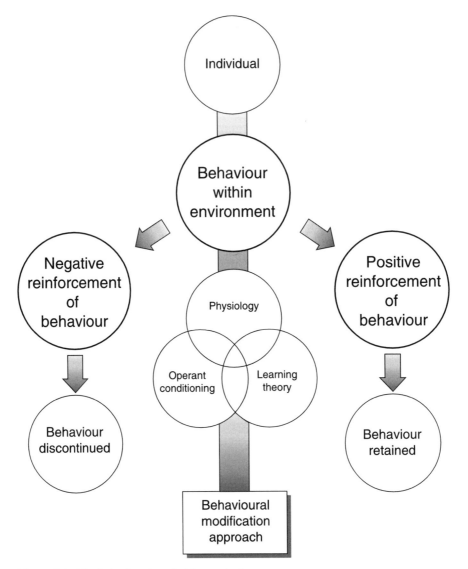

Figure 8.1 The behavioural applied frame of reference.

desired behaviour and the reward may be drawn up between patient and therapist.)

• Providing opportunities for the behaviour to occur. Prompting, shaping and cueing the behaviour if necessary.

• Providing the reward (consistently / intermittently) when the behaviour (or at first, a close approximation to it) is achieved.

• Gradually withdrawing or reducing the frequency of the reward once the behaviour has become an established part of the repertoire.

The keys to the successful use of this approach are breaking down the task, defining a clear objective, finding a reinforcer which is acceptable and effective, and, above all, a very consistent implementation of the programme by everyone involved with the patient.

Writing behavioural objectives

Writing clear behavioural objectives is an essential therapeutic skill which is often used even when not employing a behaviour modification approach. It is also a skill which is not always carried out with sufficient precision. This is mainly a matter of practice. An objective must contain both the specification of the performance and criteria by which successful completion can be measured. It is usually formed as follows:

- person (student/client)
- precise performance (define what is to be done)
- conditions (when, where, how often, how long, with/without specified form of help).

For example, the student (person) will point to the carpal bones on the skeleton and will correctly name each one (precise performance) at the first attempt and without reference to notes (conditions).

Summary of the behavioural AFR

Metamodel: Reductionist.

Origin of problem: The individual has, through faulty learning due to inappropriate reinforcement and/or environment, learnt an 'undesirable' (inappropriate, damaging, unproductive) behaviour or failed to learn a 'desirable' (appropriate, utilitarain) one.

Primary assumptions

- An individual can only be studied in terms of her observable behaviour. All actions performed by the individual are regarded as behaviour; this includes language.
- Behaviour occurs in response to stimuli which promote or decrease it.
- All behaviour is learnt. Behaviour can be unlearnt (extinguished) as well as learnt.
- Learning occurs in response to reinforcement which is either provided extrinsically by the environment or intrinsically by the behaviour. Intermittent schedules of reinforcement are the most effective.

> If you would like to practise writing behavioural objectives, try producing some for this client:
>
> Jenny is a 16-year-old girl with severe learning difficulties. She has been referred with the aim of 'improve independence in feeding'. When you visit her at lunch time you observe that she at first makes no attempt to feed herself. She is able to grasp a spoon when it is placed in her hand and rather messily tries to get some food onto it. Once she has the food in her mouth she immediately tries to get some more onto the spoon and into her mouth without leaving time for chewing and swallowing, and consequently spits out food or chokes and becomes very frustrated. She abandons her attempts at eating after a few minutes. She is very fond of music and also likes to touch a favourite cuddly toy bear.
>
> 1 Write some clear behavioural objectives for the first stage of your treatment,
> 2 Which would you tackle first? Would you work towards this in stages? If so, how might you write specific objectives for this?

- A positive reinforcer must be carefully selected to be appropriate to the individual and must be correctly and consistently used.
- Behaviour can be reduced to a simple sequence of responses: these can be taught separately if required or chained in sequence. Complex sequences combine to produce 'molar behaviour', the response of the whole organism.
- Learning programmes should be designed to meet the exact requirements of the individual.

Terminology: Behaviourism has a distinct 'language' which must be acquired to work comfortably within the approach. Frequently used terms include: patient (client); therapist; classical conditioning; operant conditioning; stimulus–response (SR) conditioning; deconditioning; extinction; positive/negative reinforcement; schedules of reinforcement; reward/punishment; time out; modelling; shaping; cueing; training; behavioural contract; behaviour modification; goal planning; behavioural objectives.

Patient/therapist relationship: In the strict form of behaviourism the patient has little to do with goal setting and need not even be capable of cooperation, the therapist controls all elements of the situation. In the more usual modified form the patient and therapist may agree a behavioural contract, or the patient may participate in goal setting.

Examples of applications:
Learning difficulties (mental handicap); skills deficits; brain injuries; psychiatric disorders: e.g. phobias, anxiety states; dependency related problems, e.g. substance abuse; behavioural problems/challenging behaviours; institutionalization.

Approach: Behaviour modification. Other techniques which may be used include: programmed learning; chaining and backward chaining; room management techniques; social modelling.

Criteria for evaluation of outcome: A previously specified behavioural performance has been observed to be consistently achieved (or a behaviour has been eliminated from the repertoire).

Advantages: Precise objectives are set, and achievement of objectives is measurable in performance terms. The associated techniques are of particular use for individuals who have moderate or severe learning difficulties, challenging behaviours or behavioural disturbances, and for people with fears originating from situational condition-

ing. Learning does not have to depend on patient motivation or cooperation. Teaching can be tailored to individual needs. Specific skills and subskills can be learnt in small stages. Behaviours can be unlearnt.

Disadvantages: Although basic behavioural theory is often used, effective application of behavioural techniques is time-consuming and must be done with great precision and expertise by all concerned; this normally requires additional training. Incorrectly applied behaviour modification is at best useless and at worst damaging. Each objective must be very carefully phrased, specifying the behaviour and the conditions under which it will be performed: if this is done 'fuzzily', therapy may be ineffective and measurement of success of dubious validity. Learning may not generalize and may fade once the reinforcement is withdrawn. The reductionist approach ignores emotional and cognitive explanations of behaviour. An overly strict application of positive/negative reinforcement, particularly if there is any element of punishment or deprivation, carries ethical implications and should be avoided.

SUGGESTED READING

Any psychology textbook will contain basic behavioural theory. The books listed under the Education Model also give good summaries of theory. Books on therapy for mentally handicapped or brain damaged individuals frequently contain information on the use of behavioural techniques.

Bandura A 1977 Social learning theory. Prentice Hall

Bigge M 1987 Learning theories for teachers, 4th edn. Harper & Row

Bruce M A, Borg B 1987 Frames of Reference in psychiatric occupational therapy. Slack, *The behavioural frame of reference*.

Gagné R M 1977 The conditions of learning and theory of instruction, 3rd edn. Holt Saunders

Jones M C 1983 Behaviour problems in handicapped children. Souvenir Press

Lovell R B 1987 Adult learning, Croom Helm

Mosey A C 1986 Psychosocial components of occupational therapy. Raven Press, *Ch. 25 & Ch. 26: the acquisitional frame of reference*.

Reed K L 1984 Models of practice in occupational therapy. Williams & Wilkins, *Ch. 6: Supermodels*.

Yule W & Carr J Behaviour modification for the mentally handicapped. Croom Helm

Willson M 1987 Occupational therapy in long-term psychiatry, 2nd edn. Churchill Livingstone, Edinburgh. *Ch. 1: Behavioural models*.

COGNITIVE-BEHAVIOURAL APPLIED FRAME OF REFERENCE

This AFR is based on the assumption that thoughts, behaviour and feelings are linked. When the individual 'feels bad' about himself or a situation this produces negative thoughts. Negative thoughts make him feel more stressed;

stress inhibits action to break out of the negative cycle. When these thoughts and feelings relate to daily activities, a cycle of dysfunction is set up in which the person feels that she can't cope, so ceases to try to do so, thus proving to herself that her original negative thought was correct — she can't cope.

There are variations on the cognitive behavioural approach, but in general it is aimed at helping the individual to:

- recognize negative emotions
- make the connection between negative emotions and negative thoughts
- see how negative thinking inhibits adaptive action
- develop challenges to negative thoughts
- replace negative thoughts with positive ones
- take control of her life by setting achievable goals and working towards these in small, successful steps
- use problem solving to reduce problems to size or find solutions
- use techniques to manage stress or improve communication with others
- reward herself for achievement.

The unconscious basis of behaviour is ignored and no attempt is made within this approach to use 'psychoanalysis' or 'psychotherapy'. The approach is firmly based in the present and looks to the future; the past is accepted but not explored. This approach is not suited to use with patients whose memory or learning abilities are impaired or who have personality disorders.

The therapist needs to assist the patient to recognize and appreciate improvements in the range of activities, quality of life, experiences of control, decisions and choices, and achievement of goals. The feedback from successful participation is very important in reinforcing changes in behaviour resulting from changes in thinking.

Summary of the cognitive-behavioural AFR

Metamodel: Organismic: thoughts, mental processes, emotions and behaviour are closely linked; input from environment affects cognition.

Origin of problem: Inability to attend; incorrect or incomplete cognitive processing, incorrect interpretation or distortion of perceptions, compulsive or negative thought processes, failure to establish an autonomous identity or to develop a positive self-concept, general misinterpretations of reality produce dysfunctions in social interactions, emotional control, cognitive strategies or ability to perform activities.

Primary assumptions
- Cognition is a complex process which may be explained by various theories.
- Each individual has a unique experience and interpretation of his environment.
- Thoughts are connected with emotions and influence behaviour; thoughts are influenced by perceptions of past and future events.
- Perceptions of self, and the way in which the individual views his past actions or plans future ones, are also governed by cognitive processes.
- Dysfunctional individuals may be helped to become functional by an analysis of cognitive processes, by improving knowledge and learning strategies, and by teaching adaptive, positive and effective cognitive strategies to replace maladaptive, negative or ineffective ones.

Terminology: Patient, client; therapist (and the language of particular techniques).

Patient/therapist relationship: Usually facilitatory.

Examples of applications
- Psychiatric disorders: e.g. anxiety, depression, obsessional states, phobias.
- Stress related disorders: e.g. chronic pain, dysfunction following disability or challenging life event, e.g. bereavement, retirement.

Approach: Cognitive behavioural.

Examples of techniques: 'homework', e.g. diary, cognitive tasks; relaxation techniques; stress management; anxiety management; assertiveness training; problem solving training; behavioural rehearsal; cognitive modelling; scripting; role-play.

Criteria for evaluation of outcome: The individual reports and/or the therapist observes improvement in cognitive skills leading to positive changes in performance and/or affect.

Advantages: Cognitive techniques generally

offer practical strategies which involve the patient in identifying the elements of her feelings/thoughts/behaviours which she wants to change and then taking action to achieve this. This is reported to produce quite rapid, observable, positive results. Interpretations of the 'unconscious' causation of behaviour are avoided and therapy may therefore be more acceptable to the patient.

Disadvantages: Some of the theoretical models or explanations of cognitive function are very complex; the techniques are based on hypotheses which cannot be 'proved' since they deal with subjective material. A great deal about the processes of cognition, and the connection between thoughts and emotions, is still conjectural.

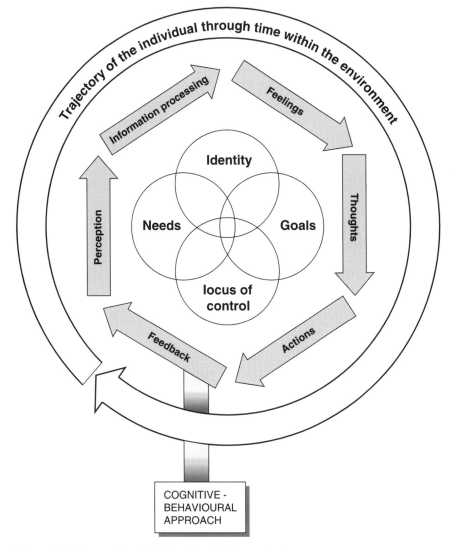

Figure 8.2 The cognitive-behavioural applied frame of reference.

SUGGESTED READING

Most psychology textbooks contain chapters on cognitive processes.
General
Creek J 1996 Occupational therapy in mental health, principles, skills and practice. Churchill Livingstone, Edinburgh. *Ch. 13*, 2nd edn: *Cognitive approaches*.
Cognitive-behavioural approach
Beck A T 1976 Cognitive therapy and the emotional disorders. Meridian, New York

Bruce M A, Borg B 1987 Frames of reference in psychiatric occupational therapy. Slack, *Cognitive frame of reference Cognitive-behavioural frame of reference*.
Dryden W, Golden W (eds) 1986 Cognitive behavioural approaches to psychotherapy. Harper and Row, London
Gross R 1992 Psychology: science of mind and behaviour, 2nd edn. Hodder and Stoughton, London
Grant L, Evans A 1994 Principles of behavioural analysis. Harper Collins College Publishers

THE ANALYTICAL APPLIED FRAME OF REFERENCE

The analytical AFR deals with the unconscious or subconscious basis of an individual's behaviour, his emotions and the personal meanings and symbolisms which he may attribute to people, events or objects. This hidden material may be uncovered by a variety of techniques. This AFR can be used with an individual in a dyadic relationship with the therapist, or with individuals loosely organized in a group.

The classical form of psychoanalysis is that originated by Freud at the beginning of the twentieth century. He created the terms which have passed into the language of analysis—e.g. unconscious, preconscious, id, ego, super-ego, libido—and proposed that the gratification of drives, especially sexuality, was the basis of human behaviour. The development of the individual during infancy and childhood follows a series of stages. Fixation in, or regression to, one of these early stages limits the development of an integrated personality.

Other schools of psychoanalysis have developed subsequently, extending or deviating from Freud's original explanations of the basis of human personality. A significant theory considers 'object relations'—the perceptions of and relationships with people or desired objects, particularly as a baby—to have a fundamental influence on subsequent relationships and behaviour.

Psychoanalysts view the individual as being motivated by unconscious drives and emotions which direct behaviour and are not subject to voluntary control. Some of these unconscious forces are innate, others arise through the interpretation of past experiences, usually as a very young child. The individual can, by a long process of analysis, during which the relationship with the analyst is a significant part of therapy, come to a better (but never complete) understanding of the reasons for his feelings and behaviour and this may help her to live a more satisfying and less anxious life. The analytical approach, therefore, takes a primarily retrospective view of human actions, understanding of the past bringing comprehension of the present and removing anxieties concerning the future.

Since Freud, many theorists have developed their own ideas following one or other of the above styles, or attempted a synthesis. The role of the analyst varies from the neutral to the directive and from the reflective to the actively interpretive or interactive. There are far too many notable names to mention them all, but some people who have produced innovatory and influential theories between the First and Second World Wars include:

- Freud (stages of sexuality; gratification of drives)
- Adler (will to power)
- Jung (dreams and symbols; archetypes and the collective unconscious)
- Klein (object relations; infantile experiences)
- Sullivan (object relations; juvenile anxiety)
- Winnicott (child/mother relationship)
- Guntrip (repressed ego).

Later theorists are even more numerous and the student is advised to read texts selectively to avoid becoming confused by elaborate and contradictory concepts.

When using this approach the occupational therapist typically uses creative and projective techniques such as art, sculpture, drama or mime, working with people as individuals or as a collection of individuals within a group. The person's reactions to and interpretation of his creative endeavours help to uncover hidden symbolisms or emotions. Discussion of these provides insight into underlying psychological mechanisms such as repression, denial, guilt, conflict or projection. This works best with intelligent, articulate patients who have a degree of insight.

Material which is brought to the surface has to be dealt with—'worked through'—so that the patient can acknowledge and cope with it. Repressed material is 'dangerous' from the patient's point of view—that is why it was repressed in the first place—it triggers uncomfortable emotions such as guilt, anxiety, sexual desires or anger, and exploration of all this can only be done, if at all, in a safe environment. This sense of trust and safety has to be created by the therapist.

Although patients may work within a group, they usually do so as individuals, not as group members. Analytical theories are concerned with the reasons for an individual's reactions to her own feelings or to other individuals or objects, not with his reactions to people in general or groups as a whole.

The degree to which an occupational therapist may interpret the use of images and symbols by the patient and the manner in which the therapist facilitates self-discovery depends on the theory within which he is working, and the techniques with which he is familiar. Sometimes it is the patient's interpretations which are used, sometimes it may be those of the therapist, but interpretations are suggested, not imposed.

The occupational therapist is not, and should not try to be, a psychoanalyst or psychotherapist. Because of the highly potent nature of unconscious material all projective techniques should be used with discretion, following suitable training, and the practitioner must have access to adaquate personal supervision. (The supervisor must be a person suitably qualified both to oversee the therapist's treatment of patients and also to deal with the dynamics of the therapist's own

needs, dilemmas and personal growth.) The material which a patient produces needs to be dealt with by a properly qualified analyst.

The approach was first developed by Fidler in the USA; she was interested in the potential of activities for releasing reactions and emotions and acting as a vehicle for communication between therapist and patient—hence her approach is sometimes called 'the communication approach'. The most frequently described approaches are: psychodynamic (analytical) approach (Levy in Willard & Spackman 1993); object relations approach (Mosey 1986).

Summary of the analytical AFR

Metamodel: Reductionist: based on the premise that a person is not capable of rational choices, behaviour being determined by the unconscious drives and past experiences and feelings which may be analysed to provide explanations of current behaviour and emotions.

Origin of problem: A deficit in or lack of integration of the personality stemming from unconscious causes. The problem is usually described within the language of a particular theory. Examples: an unresolved conflict; fixation in or regression to an early developmental stage; lack of insight; failure to acknowledge sexuality; faulty early relationship with a parent.

Primary assumptions

This summary deals with broad principles shared by the main schools of analysis as interpreted in the context of OT. In analytical practice there are marked differences between theorists which are reflected in the use of language and techniques.

- Behaviour is governed by unconscious, irrational processes, linked to the gratification of basic drives.
- Early life, during which a person develops through psychosexual stages, or stages in the development of relationships with persons and objects, has a lasting effect on personality.
- Conflicts, anxiety, guilt, depression or problems with relationships in later life are symptoms of unresolved unconscious conflicts originating in repressed memories of infancy and childhood.

- Subconscious material may surface in the form of dreams and symbols which may affect perceptions of reality.
- It is possible through a lengthy process of anlaysis to uncover the origins of symptoms, to bring material out of the unconscious, to gain insight, and thereby to resolve conflicts, anxieties and unsatisfactory relationships.

Terminology: Patient/client; analysand; therapist; analyst; therapy; analysis (and the language of the particular theorist, e.g. Freud: ego, superego, libido, transference, countertransference, projection, repression, unconscious, preconscious).

Patient/therapist relationship: It is anticipated that a complex relationship occurs during an extended process of analysis which involves mechanisms such as projection, transference and countertransference. Although the occupational therapist is not functioning as an analyst, such relationships may develop, and the therapist must be aware of his own mechanisms of defence or transference. The patient may develop some dependency on the therapist.

Examples of conditions treated: Anxiety states; affective disorders; sexual dysfunction: failure to develop a positive self-image: feelings of guilt and unworthiness; failure to develop satisfactory relationships; phobias.

Examples of approaches: Analytical (psychodynamic; Freudian/neo-Freudian); object relations.

Examples of OT techniques: Psychodrama; music therapy; guided fantasy; projective art; creative writing; mime; creative activities.

Criteria for evaluating outcome: The affective state, psychosocial function or symptoms of psychopathology experienced by the individual are observed to have improved and/or the individual reports subjective improvement.

Advantages: Focuses on emotions and relationships; releases unconscious material and makes it accessible. Recognizes an irrational basis for behaviour.

Disadvantages: Since the process is highly subjective it can be hard to define goals or the problem. The process is usually slow; results may not be apparent until months or even years after therapeutic interventions or experiences. The patient may become dependent on the therapist. Traditional Freudian thinking fosters a submissive female stereotype judged by the standards of current Western culture (neo-Freudians have modified accordingly). Psychoanalysis has not been demonstrated to be effective by objective studies (but its practitioners defend this result by saying that objective methods of research are inappropriate and impractical). For the occupational therapist, use of dynamic techniques requires expertise: overinterpretation or misinterpretation by the therapist could be misleading or damaging. Releasing unconscious material without dealing with it appropriately may produce violent emotional reactions and behaviours. Techniques may be stressful for the therapist if he uncovers personal material or emotions.

SUGGESTED READING

Books on psychoanalysis are very numerous: the best strategy is to decide which theorist you are interested in and to obtain books by, or about, him/her. Books on psychology will contain summaries of basic theory.

Balint M 1984 The basic fault. Arrowsmith, Bristol

Bruce M A, Borg B 1987 Frames of reference in psychiatric occupational therapy. Slack, New Jersey. *Object relations frame of reference.*

Creek J (ed) 1990 Occupational therapy and mental health; principles, skills and practice. Churchill Livingstone, Edinburgh. *Ch. 13: OT and group psychotherapy.*

Finlay L 1988 Occupational therapy practice in psychiatry. Croom Helm, London. *Ch. 2.*

Foulkes S H, Anthony E J 1965 Group psychotherapy: the analytical approach. Penguin, Harmondsworth

Mosey A C 1981 Configuration of a profession. Raven Press, New York. *Ch. 14: Analytical frame of reference.*

Mosey A C 1986 Psychosocial components of occupational therapy. Raven Press, New York. *Ch. 21 and Ch. 22: Analytical frame of reference.*

Reed K L 1984 Models of practice in occupational therapy. Williams & Wilkins, Baltimore. *Ch. 6: Supermodels; also Object Relations.*

Willson M 1984 Occupational therapy in short-term psychiatry, 2nd edn. Churchill Livingstone, Edinburgh

Note:

The analytical AFR and group work AFR have a similar basis and are both illustrated in Figure 8.3 in order to show this relationship.

THE GROUP WORK APPLIED FRAME OF REFERENCE

The group work AFR is based on theories concerning the dynamics of group interactions and processes and their effects on the behaviour and reactions of group members. In this AFR the group is the important entity, and all individual experiences are explored through the medium of the group. It is possible to have groups which are analytically based, but also to use other approaches, such as cognitive or humanistic, within a group setting. In occupational therapy the group may focus on some activity as a means of facilitating the group process.

In psychiatric settings there are two aspects to this AFR which may or may not overlap: firstly, a concern with the individual's skills of interpersonal communication (interactive approach/activities group approach); and, secondly, a concern with the ability of an individual to function as a member of a group, and the power of the group to function as a therapeutic entity (psychotherapeutic group approach).

The interactive/activities group approach

This form of group is structured to promote the development and use of interpersonal and social skills. The therapist will assess deficits in verbal and non-verbal communication, personal appearance and cultural appropriateness and will design situations and exercises which will promote the ability of the patient to initiate and sustain appropriate and effective interactions with other individuals, to recognize and express her own needs, and to take account of the needs of others.

This is based on cognitive and experiential methods, not behavioural ones, although the approach may also include skills training, particularly social interactive skills, communicative skills and skills in assertion. This may begin dyadically with individuals who are unable to cope with being in a group, but such techniques are most often used in a group setting where members can interact and experiment.

Mosey (1986) describes the use of activity groups in detail and lists a number of types: evaluative, task orientated, developmental and thematic. She also describes formats for developmental groups, each one involving the patient in a higher level of communication and cooperation: parallel, egocentric-cooperative, project, cooperative, mature.

The choice of activity and the arrangement of the environment in which the group takes place are crucial in promoting the right level of interaction.

The psychotherapeutic group approach

Group therapy is based on theories of group dynamics and may borrow or adapt techniques derived from psychotherapeutic practice. There is a wide spectrum of types of groups, from relatively unstructured, open groups to closed psychotherapy groups which operate over an extended period with a fixed number of participants, and which may or may not involve task related activity.

It is typical of this form of group work that the product of group activity, whilst giving the group a focus and a potential sense of achievement, is subordinate to the group process, which provides the insights and learning experiences for group members and gives the therapist opportunities to explore both individual issues and group dynamics.

There may be a degree of interpretation and analysis of the dynamics of interactions, or the results of participation in activities, but often the main purpose of the group is to provide opportunities for patients to participate in order to explore their personal reactions and problems by means of interactions and shared group processes or to improve their abilities to communicate their own needs and to be sensitive to those of others.

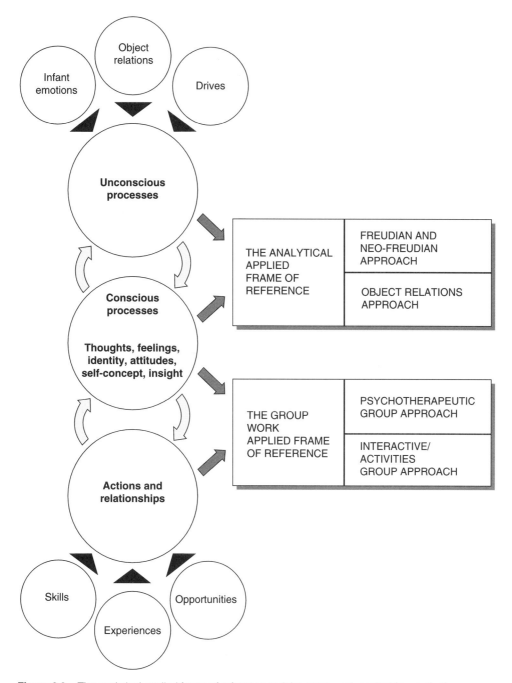

Figure 8.3   The analytical applied frame of reference and the group work applied frame of reference.

The role of the therapist in facilitating this process, and the style of leadership used, are crucial. A group takes time to form, to reach a point where members function as a group and not as individuals, and even longer to reach a point where it really 'performs'. Therapeutic groups are essentially artificial creations and can be difficult to manage—there is a great deal of scope for conflict, the group may disintegrate, split into 'cliques', or get sidelined away from important issues. A therapist needs to be very experienced and knowledgeable about group theory and group techniques to manage conflicts constructively and get the best out of a group. A 'good' group is cohesive, mutually supportive, goal orientated and productive. When a group really does 'gel' the results can be exciting.

Summary of the group work AFR

Metamodel: This AFR tends to be undogmatic. In the sense that it is more concerned with the individual's perceptions of reality and reactions to and communication with others it is holistic, but analysis may also be carried out. There is often a pragmatic (if philosophically unsound) synthesis of ideas and techniques which accepts both metamodels as valid.

Origin of problem: Because of past bad experiences, lack of opportunities, lack of skills, psychiatric disorder or faulty perceptions of reality, the individual is unable to identify or to express her own needs and wishes, to form relationships, to communicate with others or to take account of the needs and wishes of others.

Primary assumptions
- The skills of interacting with other people can only be acquired experientially.
- Interaction with other people in structured therapeutic groups provides a means of achieving personal growth and insight and developing interactive skills.
- The group process is in itself a dynamic and potent therapeutic medium.
- Personal growth is a painful process which requires a secure and supportive group environment.
- Group work can facilitate communication and cohesion between group members and provides a means of dealing with conflicts.

Terminology: Client; therapist; co-therapist; group leader; facilitator; closed group; open group; group process; group dynamic; activity group.

Examples of applications: Group techniques are used with a great variety of people, e.g. staff groups, support groups, carers groups, as well as for the treatment of psychiatric conditions. Group work is not normally used with people who are highly disturbed, hyperactive, have personality disorders (psychopaths) or produce very challenging or disruptive behaviour.

Approaches: Interactive/activities group; psychotherapeutic group.

Examples of techniques
- Interactive approach
  — social activities
  — social games, quizzes etc.
  — group projects
  — creative activities
  — role-play
  — social/communication skills training
- psychotherapeutic approach
  — 'role-play'
  — 'gaming'
  — projective techniques
  — psychodrama
  — assertion training
  — anxiety management
  — stress management
  — communication skills training
  — social skills training.

Criteria for evaluating outcome: The individual shows improved awareness of herself and others and improved abilities to express her own needs and meet those of others.

Advantages: When well led or facilitated, group work can produce good results. Working with people in groups is an effective use of resources. The group process is experiential and highly relevant to the client; although beneficial results may be slow to appear they tend to be long-lasting.

Disadvantages: A group needs to meet several times to be effective. A psychotherapeutic group may need to continue for several months and results may not appear until long after the group is ended. Group management—whichever style of leadership or facilitation is employed—is highly skilled. Group work is stressful for the therapist, who must have access to proper supervision. Although psychoanalysis is not usually the main purpose, group processes can produce unexpected and potentially explosive reactions if material surfaces unexpectedly, and this must be correctly dealt with. Psychotherapeutic groups which involve no 'occupational' element do not require the use of OT primary core skills. A group may become a vehicle for 'talking therapy' which produces little result.

SUGGESTED READING

Creek J (ed) 1996 Occupational therapy and mental health; principles, skills and practice. Churchill Livingstone, Edinburgh. *Ch. 14:* Groupwork, 2nd edn

Gerard B A, Boniface W J, Howe B H 1980 Interpersonal skills for health professionals. Reston, Virginia

Heap K 1979 Process and action in working with groups. Pergamon Press, Oxford

Hopkins H L, Smith H D (eds) 1993 Willard & Spackman's occupational therapy, 8th edn. Lippincott, Philadelphia. *Section 2: Group process.*

Howe M C, Shwartzenburg S L 1986 A functional approach to group work in occupational therapy. Lippincott, Philadelphia

Mosey A C 1986 Psychosocial components of occupational therapy. Raven Press, New York. *Chs 12, 13, 14: Groups.*

Kielhofner G 1992 Conceptual foundations of occupational therapy. F A Davis, Philadelphia. *Ch. 9: Group work.*

Reed K L 1984 Models of practice in occupational therapy. Williams & Wilkins, Baltimore. *Ch. 13: Intra and interpersonal performance. Models.*

Remocker A J, Storch E T 1982 Action speaks louder. Churchill Livingstone, Edinburgh

Robertson E 1984 The role of the occupational therapist in a psychotherapeutic setting. British Journal of Occupational Therapy 47(4)

Willson M 1984 Occupational therapy in short-term psychiatry. Churchill Livingstone, Edinburgh

Yallom I D 1975 Theory and practice of group psychotherapy. Basic Books, New York

Yallom I D 1983 In-patient group psychotherapy. Basic Books, New York

Whittaker D S 1985 Using groups to help people. Routledge & Kegan, London

THE HUMANISTIC APPLIED FRAME OF REFERENCE

The basis of humanism and its relevance to OT has been explained in Chapter 6. The humanistic AFR has given rise to two approaches:

- client centred approach
- student centred approach.

These are based on a very similar set of ideas, but the former is used in a therapeutic setting, and the latter in an educational one.

The client centred approach

In this approach the client is encouraged to direct her own therapy as far as may be possible, to accept personal responsibility and to make decisions. Aims of treatment and activities are selected by the client and must have some personal meaning for her. The development of a sense of self-worth, and an internal locus of control are seen as important.

The therapist acts as a facilitator, offering opportunities, enabling the client to explore thoughts and feelings in a safe environment, and providing resources which the client identifies as necessary.

Validation of personal perceptions and experiences is important, but the therapist may help the client to question or challenge aspects of her life with which she is dissatisfied. Sometimes a mutual contract is agreed which sets the boundaries for intervention. Where a client is incapable of making her own choices, the therapist, or another person, acts as her advocate, putting forward her wishes in so far as they can be ascertained and attempting to put the client's viewpoint as she might have done herself.

The client centred approach is not occupationally based, and in order to provide a more distinct OT focus it has been developed into an OT model (the Canadian client centred model) which is described in Section 4.

The student centred approach

The learner is expected to be pro-active in setting personal goals and finding means to achieve

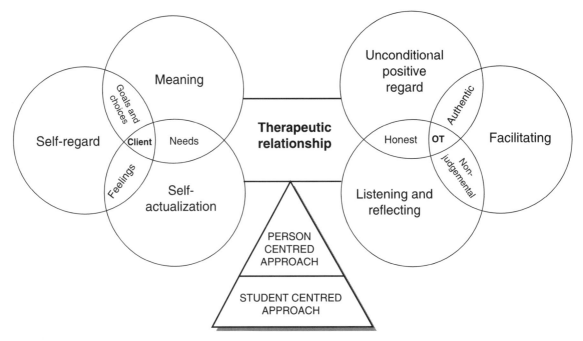

Figure 8.4 The humanistic applied frame of reference.

these. The therapist (in the role of teacher) again acts as a facilitator, providing resources, discussing the results of learning, helping the student to formulate goals, explore concepts and test ideas.

Summary of the humanistic AFR

Metamodel: Strongly holistic.

Origin of problem: The individual is dysfunctional because of damage, developmental disorder, lack of opportunity to acquire skill, lack of the information required to make correct choices, environmental stress, failure to achieve; poor self-actualization, lack of positive regard from others, poor self-esteem, or a combination of such factors.

Primary assumptions

• The personal experience and consciousness of the individual is of paramount importance; since no one else can experience it, no one should attempt to influence another's choices or interpretations of reality.

• The individual must be considered as a whole in the context of his physical and social environment.

• An individual has the right to personal choice (and all other human rights).

• The goal of the individual is to be autonomous, authentic and self-actualizing (functioning as a free, self-directing, honest person whose life brings self-satisfaction and contains personal meaning).

• The individual is capable of controlling events in her life and should direct her own education or therapy as far as possible.

• An individual is innately capable of positive development.

Terminology: Client; facilitator; counsellor; person centred therapy; counselling; self-directed learning, autheticity; self-actualization.

Client/therapist relationship: Central to this approach is the rejection of power being exercised by one person over another. Therapy must be client centred and the therapist must ensure that control is given to the client, even at the expense of very slow decision-taking. The therapist acts as facilitator, providing opportunities and information to enable the client to decide what she wants and then arranging the resources, or intervention, to achieve this.

Examples of application: Can be used with any individual.

Approaches: Person centred; student centred.

Examples of associated OT techniques: Counselling; group work and role-play; client centred rehabilitation or education; assertion training; creative therapies; guided fantasy; psychodrama; relaxation; yoga; meditation.

Although the therapist may select techniques which facilitate the client's opportunities for choice and self-expression, if the client is temporarily, or by nature of her dysfunction, unable to do so, selection of techniques should normally be negotiated between the client and the therapist, or selected by the client.

Criteria for evaluation of outcome: The client accepts that whatever outcomes she set for herself or negotiated with the therapist have been achieved, or that the need for the therapist's intervention has ended.

Advantages: As a general philosophy of care it is widely applicable. It is a dynamic, holistic, flexible approach which can deal with psychological, developmental and physical dysfunction, and with deteriorating and terminal conditions. As a method of counselling or teaching the process is client directed and it is therefore perceived as highly relevant, motivation is positive and results tend to be permanent.

Disadvantages: It can be slow, goals can be 'fuzzy', it may, if taken too literally, be so nondirective that nothing happens and the process can be 'all talk, no do'. This approach may not be comfortably compatible with the central 'occupations and activities' concerns of occupational therapy, in which case the client would be better referred to a counsellor. The concept of a person being able to control all the choices in her life may be overstated and unrealistic. Interventions can be hard to evaluate so that evidence of success is often anecdotal.

SUGGESTED READING

There is a large amount of literature and you need to track down books by the theorist in whom you are interested. Because the philosophy of humanism is closely related to that of occupational therapy, some books discussing theory are listed below in addition to the OT references.

Abraham B 1988 The dilemmas of helping someone towards independence: an experiential account. British Journal of Occupational Therapy

Eagan G 1986 The skilled helper. Brooks Cole, California.

Finlay L 1988 Occupational therapy practice in psychiatry. Croom Helm, London. *Ch. 2*

Kirshenbaun H, Henderson V L (eds) 1990 Carl Rogers dialogues. Constable, London

Maslow A H 1968 Towards a psychology of being. Van Nostrad, New York

Maslow A H 1970 Motivation and personality. Harper & Row, New York

Rogers C 1984 Client centred therapy: its current practice, implications and theory. Houghton Miffin, Boston

Rogers C 1986 On becoming a person. Constable

Willson M 1984 Occupational therapy in short-term psychiatry. Churchill Livingstone, Edinburgh. *Ch. 4: Humanistic psychology.*

Willson M 1987 Occupational therapy in long-term psychiatry. Churchill Livingstone, Edinburgh. *Ch. 2: Humanistic influence.*

9

Processes of change

DEVELOPMENT, EDUCATION, REHABILITATION AND ADAPTATION

From the moment an individual is born he becomes subject to processes of change. Changes occur as part of normal growth, maturation and ageing, and as a response to the demands of the physical or social environment and the challenges of living. Without change normal life is impossible. Basic survival depends on it. The human ability to continue to have a fulfilled and varied life, adopting or discarding roles and occupations, changing relationships, developing interests and meeting challenges throughout all the stages of living is fundamentally dependent on being able to change.

Change may occur gradually, almost unnoticed, but often change is experienced as difficult, stressful, threatening or uncomfortable, especially when it is imposed by circumstances which appear beyond one's control, whether these are due to the changes of maturation and ageing, or to external circumstances such as stressful life events including illness, bereavement, redundancy and divorce. Even pleasant events such as moving into a home of one's own, marriage, having children or being promoted require personal change.

When faced with stressful change the ability to cope or recover may depend on the degree to which the person can alter in response to these adverse circumstances. Someone who is fixed in rigid patterns of thought or behaviour can only react to things as they used to be, not as they now are. Such a person never manages to move away from loss, grief, physical limitation, or personal disappointment. He is confined within limitations of his own making and by routines and habits which persist and are resistant to adaptation.

Every therapist rapidly becomes aware that the person who is positive, adaptive and flexible has a far better chance of living a fulfilling and satisfying life, even in the face of great difficulties or disabilities, compared to the non-adaptive person whose problems may be less challenging.

Occupational therapy is itself a process of 'changing through doing'. The principles of occupational therapy have been derived from the theoretical and scientific background of several of the fundamental processes of change, human development, human learning, and human adaptation. Rehabilitation evolved as a synthesis of physical and psychosocial therapies aimed at achieving constructive change and recovery following illness or injury, and adapting to or compensating for the effects of residual disability.

As described in Chapter 4, these processes are hard to classify because they operate at various levels; each is large and complex enough to be described as a paradigm in its own right. They are also quite closely interlinked.

Studies of learning and development have given rise to much theory building and model making, with associated approaches. These have influenced the theories and practices of rehabilitation. As interpreted by various professions in education and health care, they have generated further applied frames of reference and approaches. Adaptation has elements of all the other three, plus a strong influence from systems theory, and from the practice of occupational therapy.

Development, education and adaptation are closely linked, but it is helpful to separate them. *Development* relates to the predetermined sequence in which maturation takes place, and also to the active use of innate potential which an individual has for learning.

Education is concerned with the physiological, cognitive and affective changes which are required if learning is to take place, with the effects of environment on learning, and with teaching techniques which promote learning.

Adaptation is 'individual adjustment or change made by a person to enhance survival and potential of that individual' (Reed & Sanderson 1992). It concerns the capacity of the individual to interpret the environment accurately and then to make appropriate responses to it, and the capacity to retain the most useful and adaptive responses and to discard ones which are not adaptive.

Each of these processes has helped to influence and shape the philosophy and practice of occupational therapy and has been incorporated into the theory base of applied frames of reference and OT practice models. Occupational therapy is concerned with the individual as a skilled and competent performer of a range of roles and occupations appropriate to his age, environment and culture; each process contributes in some way to the attainment and retention of skilled performance.

Summary: processes of change

- **Development**: Produces change through maturation and by active use of the potentials which build complex skills.
- **Education**: Produces change through the acquisition of knowledge, skills and attitudes which are incorporated into daily life.
- **Rehabilitation**: Produces change which operates to restore function and independence following illness or injury.
- **Adaptation**: Produces useful change which enables a person to respond to the demands of daily life and to enhance and maintain well-being.

It is important for a therapist to identify which of these processes is most significant for her patient. One cannot, for example, rehabilitate — restore — a skill which was never there to begin with; if the skill was not there it must be trained. One cannot train someone to use a skill if the prerequisite developmental potential is not present or if the required developmental level has not been attained. A person who cannot learn (attend to, perceive, store and recall information and relate this to his situation) cannot adapt. It is, therefore, important that the student understands the scope of these processes and their relationship to occupational therapy.

Adaptation, in particular, is viewed as a central part of OT Philosophy.

Adaptation is a change in function that promotes survival and self-actualization. Biological, psychological and environmental factors may interrupt the adaptation process at any time throughout the life cycle. Dysfunction may occur when adaptation is impaired. Purposeful activity facilitates the adaptive process. Occupational therapy is based on the belief that purposeful activity (occupation) including its interpersonal and environmental components, may be used to prevent and mediate dysfunction and to elicit maximum adaptation (AJOT 1995 49 (10) 1026: statement of the philosophical base of occupational therapy).

Occupational therapy is concerned with the individual as a skilled and competent performer of a range of roles and occupations appropriate to his age, environment and culture; each process contributes in some way to the attainment and retention of skilled performance.

DEVELOPMENT

Development is usually described as a hierarchical process in which one stage has to be completed before the next. The first 18 or so years of human life follow a genetically programmed developmental sequence leading to maturation. Developmental stages are innate, and each person is born with a finite and predetermined package of potential. If the potential for performance is not there, nothing can be done about it, but the extent to which potential, however large or small, is turned into competent performance depends on environmental influences and opportunities to learn, discover, experiment, practise and gain experience.

The 'nature v. nurture' debate remains unresolved: in the past decade environmental influences have been emphasized, but recent studies comparing identical twins reared in differing environments suggest that genetic factors may be more important than previously thought,

providing the potential for skills and, more controversially, even interests and preferences.

There does appear to be agreement that environment remains the most important factor; a person with the potential for genius would be profoundly limited if raised in an environment where there was a total absence of stimulation or conversation, whereas a person with severe learning difficulties would be able to make the best possible use of limited potential given individual attention and a richly stimulating environment.

Educationally, developmental theory is of use in looking at the way children learn and acquire skills (motor, perceptual, cognitive, social) (Piaget). In the context of adult learning, theories deal more with the sequence in which cognitive abilities and concepts are developed and refined (e.g. Perry, Bruner).

Physiologically, developmental theories are concerned with the maturation of the central nervous system and the sequence of acquisition of neuromuscular control, proprioceptive discrimination and perceptual skills. Incomplete, retarded or dysfunctional development is very significant to the therapist since a person cannot perform in a manner for which he is developmentally unready.

Psychosocial developmental theories look at stages in the maturation of the individual's personality and self-concept.

Summary of the development process

Metamodel: Apart from the deterministic aspects of genetic inheritance, the model is holistic, viewing the individual as a complex organism in whom all parts are interrelated, and on whom the environment also has an influence.

Origin of problem: Dysfunction is due to incomplete, retarded or maladaptive development, or to the effects of stress or trauma which may have caused the individual to regress to a more primitive developmental level (stress = regress).

Primary assumptions
• All individuals have developmental potential.

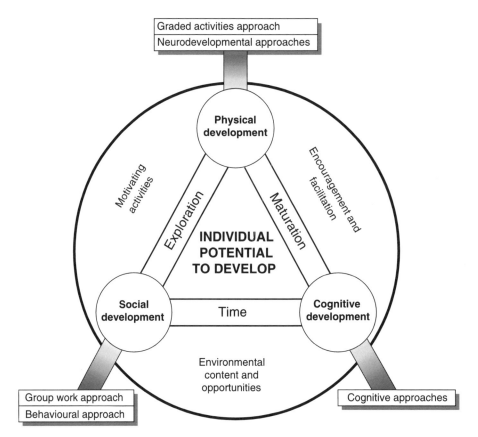

Figure 9.1 The process of development.

- The individual develops (physically, intellectually, emotionally, socially) in a defined sequence related to age.
- Stages in the developmental sequence cannot be missed or jumped if the individual is to function within the norms for his age/developmental level.
- The individual cannot function at a higher level than his stage of development. (But some authorities accept that it is possible to develop unevenly, and to be mature in some respects but not in others.)
- Environment, experience and opportunity limits, or maximizes, the extent to which developmental potential can be fulfilled.
- Development is achieved by the integration of responses through practice, experiment, and exploration; the therapist can facilitate development by reinforcing responses, aiding

integration and creating the opportunities for practice and exploration.

Terminology: Therapist; patient/client; function/dysfunction; developmental sequence/levels; therapy; intervention.

Patient/therapist relationship: This is affected by the age and degree of dysfunction of the patient, and there is a wide continuum, from the therapist being strongly controlling and directive to a partnership between therapist and patient. Because the therapist has to work within a developmental framework which implies setting quite precise objectives for therapy, some degree of prescriptive control is inevitable.

Examples of Applications: Psychiatric disorders; neurological disorders; sensorimotor disorders; learning difficulties; paediatric disorders.

Examples of Associated approaches: Neurodevelopmental (Bobath; Rood; PNF; Conductive Education); cognitive disabilities (Alan); sensory integration (Ayres); spatiotemporal; facilitating growth and development (Llorens); development of adaptive skills; recapitulation of ontogenesis (Mosey).

Techniques: Those associated with the above approaches.

Criteria for evaluation of outcome: The individual has achieved the normal developmental level for his/her age/sex or has shown progression from one level to a more advanced one.

Advantages: The process of development is based on well-researched physiological, psychological and learning theories. Developmental approaches are optimistically progressive, and can benefit people with low abilities and severe learning deficits, as well as those who have regressed to a lower developmental level as a result of illness, trauma or stress.

Disadvantages: Working developmentally can be slow and usually requires intensive therapy. The therapist must be confident and thoroughly competent when working neurodevelopmentally where effective application requires expert use of techniques which take practice and experience, and a sound comprehension of the basic theory. Progress can be retarded or lost unless all members of the team use the same techniques consistently. This model is not appropriate for deteriorating or terminal conditions (although some of the associated techniques may be) and may not be appropriate for elderly people.

SUGGESTED READING

Bruce M A, Borg B 1987 Frames of reference in psychiatric occupational therapy. Slack, New Jersey. *Developmental frame of reference.*

Hopkins H L, Smith H D (eds) 1993 Willard & Spackman's Occupational Therapy. Lippincott, Philadelphia. *Ch. 4: Section 3D Developmental F of R Section 3E Neurodevelopmental Section 3F Sensory integration F of R. Ch. 5: Section 2a and 2b human development.*

Mosey A C 1986 Psychosocial components of occupational therapy. Raven Press, New York. *Ch. 5 Age: the life cycle. Ch. 23: Developmental frame of reference. Ch. 24: Recapitulation of ontogensis.*

Reed K L 1984 Models of practice in occupational therapy. Williams & Wilkins, Baltimore. *Developmental, neurodevelopmental and neuroperceptual models.*

Willson M 1987 Occupational therapy in long-term psychiatry. Churchill Livingstone, Edinburgh. *Ch. 4: Developmental Approaches.*

THE PROCESS OF EDUCATION

Some therapists say firmly that occupational therapists are *therapists* not *teachers*. That is true, but it would clearly be misleading to say that therapists do not teach: many spend much of their time doing so, but often in an informal, unstructured manner, which may be so subliminal that both therapist and client fail to recognize the process. Mosey (1986) acknowledges that this has been so, but she has no doubts that 'the teaching-learning process has been a tool of occupational therapy since its inception'.

OT involvement in education can at other times be more formal and readily identifiable. Education of colleagues, other professions, health education for the general public, teaching specific skills, student education and supervision are important and integral parts of the therapist's role.

Perhaps some of the misunderstandings arise from the fact that the therapist deals mainly (paediatrics excepted) with adult learners — a fact which has been called *andragogy* (Knowles 1978) as distinct from pedagogy. Moreover, the therapist frequently deals with adults who have special learning needs. There has been considerable research into adult learning styles and appropriate methods of teaching adults, the more recent of which tend to emphasize the importance of moving towards student centred and experiential styles of learning, rather than teacher centred instruction. Except in the case of special needs or remedial teaching, where the edges between therapist and teacher truly blur, the therapist usually has a different basis for the use of educational techniques, and differing concerns from those of the teacher.

Theories of learning and the related teaching techniques are derived from the primary frames of reference previously discussed:

- Physiological: researching into the neurophysiology of learning.
- Behavioural: breaking down complex behaviour into skills and subskills and viewing learning as a product of environmental reward and reinforcement.
- Cognitive: viewing learning as dependent on cognitive processes; (remembering, processing, storing, retrieving) which then direct behaviour, and cognitive-developmental, looking at the sequences in which various skills are learnt.
- Social: seeing learning as linked to our perceptions of others and their behaviours.
- Humanistic: emphasizing that one cannot teach another person, only facilitate his experiential self-directed learning.

One of the few things on which the opposing theorists agree is that learning is fundamental to human behaviour. The debate over how one should define learning, or behaviour, how an individual learns, what is learnt, or which is the best method of ensuring that learning takes place, has filled many educational textbooks.

A definition of learning is 'the relatively permanent changes in potential for performance that result from past interactions with the environment'. (Lovell 1986). Learning is distinguished from changes due to basic physical maturation, although the individual has to learn in order to make best use of the potentials which come with each stage of maturation.

What is learnt can be divided into knowledge, skills and attitudes. Therapists often need to increase a person's knowledge, improve his skills or change his attitudes. Another distinction is between declarative knowledge (being able to say what you know) and procedural knowledge (being able to demonstrate you can do something). Researchers have studied differing learning styles or strategies, e.g. atomist v. holist; surface v. deep.

Educational theorists discuss the differences between these types of learning, and suggest differing ways of teaching in different circumstances. There are many similarities between the process of education — requiring aims, objectives and methods of achieving these — and the process of therapy.

In view of the amount of time therapists spend attempting to produce 'relatively permanent changes in potential for performance' it is surprising to find that few OT textbooks spend much, if any, space on educational theory as such. One has to scan the indexes and read selectively. There is, on the other hand, an overwhelming amount of educational literature.

Summary of the process of education

Metamodel: The process of education can be either holistic or reductionist, depending on the approach being used.

Origin of problem: The client/patient/learner has failed to learn because of: a cognitive deficit; a learning difficulty; lack of opportunity, experience or instruction. Inadequate, incomplete or incorrect learning results in a lack of knowledge or of skill, or an inappropriate attitude or behaviour, leading to deficits in performance.

Primary assumptions
- Most human behaviour is learnt (but there are various theoretical explanations of the way in which this occurs).
- Effective learning results in a long-lasting change in behaviour.
- It is possible to improve knowledge or skills or to develop attitudes by providing appropriate teaching, practice or experience.
- Given time and the right techniques, all but the most severely brain damaged individuals are capable of some learning.

Terminology: Client/patient/student/learner/trainee. Therapist/trainer/teacher/instructor. Teaching/training/instructing/demonstrating/educating. Learning objectives; skills; competencies.

Learner/therapist relationship: Reductionist approaches: the therapist controls and directs; the student learns, actively or passively. Holistic/

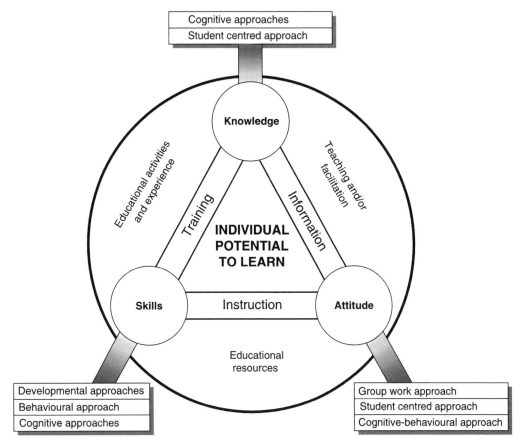

Figure 9.2 The process of education.

humanistic approaches: student centred — the therapist facilitates, teaches; the student learns actively and may direct the whole process.
Examples of Educational approaches: Physiological; behavioural; cognitive-perceptual; cognitive-behavioural; social; student centred.

Examples of Techniques
- Physiological, e.g. training motor skills and perceptual-motor skills; biofeedback.
- Behavioural, e.g. behavioural modification; errorless learning; chaining and backward chaining; habit training.
- Cognitive-perceptual, e.g. memory and perceptual training.
- Cognitive-behavioural, e.g. cognitive restructuring; anxiety management; assertion training.

- Cognitive-developmental, e.g. conductive education; portage.
- Social, e.g. social modelling; role-play; social skills training.
- Humanistic, e.g. student centred learning; experiential learning.

Criteria for evaluating outcome: Learning objectives have been met: there is observed to be a permanent change in the individual's knowledge, skill or attitude as a result of new learning.
Advantages/disadvantages: Methods and contexts are so varied that a brief discussion of advantages and disadvantages is impossible. Possibly the main disadvantage is that any learning process takes time and learners experiencing difficulties require a large amount of individual attention if learning is to be effective.

SUGGESTED READING

These publications are particularly helpful to a therapist, and deal with adult learning. If you wish to pursue this topic further, you will find many more references in the books.

Bandura A 1977 Social learning theory. Prentice Hall

Bigge M 1987 Learning theories for teachers, 4th edn. Harper & Row, New York

Gagné R M 1977 The conditions of learning and theory of instruction, 3rd edn. Holt Saunders (Cognitive/ behavioural approach)

Lovell R B 1987 Adult Learning. Croom Helm, London (basic review of theories)

Mocellin G 1988 A perspective on the principles and practice of occupational therapy. British Journal of Occupational Therapy (JAN)

Mosey A C 1986 Psychosocial components of occupational therapy. Raven Press, New York. *Ch. 9: The teaching-learning process*

Rogers C 1993 Freedom to learn for the 80s. Bell & Howell

Watts N T 1990 Handbook of clinical teaching. Churchill Livingstone, Edinburgh (Subtitled exercises and guidelines for health professionals who teach patients, train staff or supervise students.)

THE PROCESS OF REHABILITATION

Rehabilitation has been defined by the World Health Organization as: 'the combined and coordinated use of medical, social, educational and vocational measures for training or retraining the individual to the highest possible level of functional ability' (WHO 1974).

The overlap with education is plain, indeed, rehabilitation is sometimes called re-education. The root of the word is the Latin *habilitas*, meaning deftness or skill, so the word means literally, 'reskill'.

WHO further distinguishes between medical, social and vocational rehabilitation, as follows:

- **Medical rehabilitation**. The process of medical care aiming at developing the functional and psychological abilities of the individual and if necessary his compensatory mechanisms, so as to enable him to attain self-dependence and lead an active life.
- **Social rehabilitation**. That part of the rehabilitation process aimed at the integration or reintegration of a disabled person into society by helping him to adjust to the demands of family, community and occupation while reducing any economic or social burdens that may impede the total rehabilitation process.
- **Vocational rehabilitation**. The provision of those vocational services, e.g. vocational guidance, vocational training and selective placement, designed to enable a disabled person to secure and retain suitable employment (WHO 1974).

In these definitions medical and social rehabilitation clearly involve an element of adaptation — the person needs to adjust to, and compensate for, his difficulties.

In British practice the rehabilitation process is still one of the most widely used formats for therapy and the majority of British OT textbooks on physical disabilities written before 1980 have primarily been based upon it (Jones 1964; McDonald 1964; Jones & Jay 1977).

The aims of rehabilitation are well defined:

- To enable the individual to achieve independence in the areas of work and self-care.
- To restore the individual's functional ability to the previously attained level or as close to this as possible.
- To maximize and maintain the potential of retained, undamaged abilities.
- To compensate for residual disbility by means of aids, appliances, orthoses or environmental adaptations.

The process of rehabilitation requires a detailed knowledge of the patient's medical, social and environmental circumstances: aims of treatment must be geared closely to the needs of the individual. Methods include use of techniques drawn from the biomechanical, neurodevelopmental, cognitive, behavioural, group work and, more recently, client centred approaches.

As implied by the WHO definition, rehabilitation is normally viewed as an interdisciplinary process in which members of a team bring together skills appropriate to the needs of the patient and work in close cooperation to achieve jointly agreed rehabilitative goals, normally under medical direction.

The strongest focuses of physical rehabilitation have traditionally been on the restoration of sensorimotor function, independence in activities of daily living (ADL), work skills and social skills. Rehabilitation is also used as a model in psychiatry, particularly in preparation for return to community care of people who have become institutionalized and deskilled through very long stays in hospital or the effects of severe psychotic illness.

However, there has formerly been a tendency to regard the patient as being 'prescribed' rehabilitation, rather in the way that he may be prescribed a pill and then be expected to 'keep taking the tablets'. In this 'medical model' of rehabilitation the patient is expected to comply with the advice of the doctor and rehabilitation team and to work towards his recovery in the manner suggested and with relatively little opportunity to influence the process.

More recently a social model of disability has been proposed which emphasizes the necessity of society learning to accept and adjust to the needs of disabled individuals so that basic rights which apply to non-disabled people—equal opportunities for work, leisure, access to buildings, travel—are automatically available to the disabled members of society, just as they are for everyone else. In this model the person with a disability is placed in the pivotal role of expressing his needs and obtaining from professionals the services he wants and values, rather than those which they feel he 'ought' to have. This perspective has been influential in making rehabilitation into a more client centred process.

Summary of the process of rehabilitation

Metamodel: The model is nominally holistic, and the importance of taking a broadly based view of the patient and his needs, and of considering ability as well as disability is often stressed in the literature. It has to be admitted, however, that in practice, probably because of its long association with the medical model and because of the constraints on available treatment time, the model can become reductionist, homing in on the lost function and excluding the wider issues. This is particularly so in fast-flow physical rehabilitation when using a biomechanical approach.

Origin of the problem: The patient has lost a previous ability (abilities) due to illness or trauma.

Primary assumptions
- Therapy should promote personal independence and should restore function to the previous level or near 'normal'.
- Restoration of function can be achieved by graded practice of the damaged ability.
- Retraining should be carried out under realistic conditions with a view to the eventual resettlement location, social situation or work of the patient.
- Where residual disability persists, this may be compensated for by teaching the patient new skills or through the provision of aids, appliances, environmental adaptations or assistance from someone else.

Terminology: Therapist; patient (client when in the community); ability/disability; handicap; impairment; dependence/independence; therapy; treatment; restoration; re-education; resettlement; rehabilitation.

Patient/therapist relationship: The patient must actively cooperate and be involved in his rehabilitation: the success of rehabilitation is dependent on the skill with which the therapist can build a therapeutic relationship and motivate the patient to participate. Although this relationship is a partnership, traditionally the therapist tends to be the controlling partner, prescribing, advising and providing resources (another legacy of the medical model). However, a humanistic attitude is becoming more common, encouraging the client/patient to direct the rehabilitation process and to select and prioritize personal goals.

Application: The rehabilitation model can be used to treat physical illness or injury or psychiatric illness.

Examples of Associated approaches: Biomechanical; compensatory (later stages of recovery); neurodevelopmental (early stages of

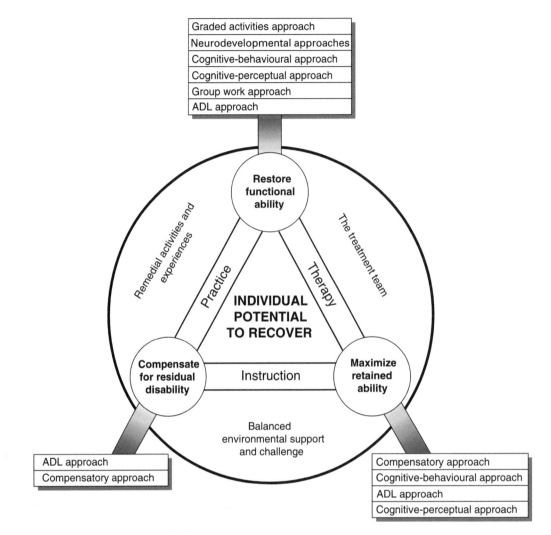

Figure 9.3 The process of rehabilitation.

recovery); cognitive perceptual; behavioural; group work.

Examples of Associated techniques: One of the strengths of the model is that it is compatible with many techniques: the danger is that too many techniques may be combined at one time, thus leading to therapeutic inconsistency. For example, it would not be effective to combine biomechanical and neurodevelopmental techniques in physical rehabilitation (if you are still not sure why, see box 7.1, p. 75). Because rehabilitation evolved early in the history of professional practice it is also closely associated with the core skills of the profession, particularly assessment, adaptation of occupations, activities and tasks and environmental adaptation.

Examples of Specific techniques
- Physical rehabilitation
  — assessment and retraining of activities of daily living
  — provision of aids and home adaptations
  — graded physical/cognitive/perceptual rehabilitation programmes (using biomechanical, cognitive or neurodevelopmental approaches)

— specific prescription of remedial activities
— work retraining and resettlement
— prescription and provision of orthoses
— prosthetic training
• Psychiatric rehabilitation
— assessment of social and self-care skills
— social skills training
— behavioural modification
— specific activities to redevelop cognitive, social, self-care or creative skills
— industrial therapy, work retraining and resettlement
— preparation for community living (group homes and hostels).

Criteria for evaluation of outcome: The lost function has been demonstrated to be restored to normal and/or a satisfactory method of compensating for residual disability has been found. The patient has been resettled in a normal, or adapted, domestic and/or work environment.

Advantages: A positive approach, aiming to improve necessary abilities, maximize existing function and compensate for deficits. Highly practical and good at problem solving. A valuable, well understood, team approach.

Disadvantages: Because of its innately optimistic assumption of improvement, this process is less applicable to deteriorating, chronic or terminal conditions. It is also inapplicable in the context of learning disorders, since here it is a matter of 'habilitation', and the other processes are more appropriate. There may be a tendency to focus on the lost abilities, rather than on those which still exist. If application is allowed to become reductionist only the obvious problems may be tackled, perhaps dealing with effects rather than causes or failing to take account of psychological problems in a physical setting: skills tend to be dealt with rather than roles or relationships. If overly prescriptive, the patient may be pressed to comply with action which is not his first choice. However, the fact that this model has stood the test of time better than most indicates that it has relatively few disadvantages.

SUGGESTED READING

Creek J (ed) 1996 Occupational therapy and mental health: principles, skills and practice, 2nd edn. Churchill Livingstone, Edinburgh. *Ch. 19: Long term client groups; Ch. 20: Rehabilitation*
Goodwill C J, Chamberlain M A (eds) 1988 Rehabilitation of the physically disabled adult. Croom Helm, London
Turner A (ed) 1996 Occupational therapy and physical dysfunction, 4th edn. Churchill Livingstone, Edinburgh

Watts F, Bennett D (eds) 1981 Principles of psychiatric rehabilitation. Wiley, Chichester
Willson M 1984 Occupational therapy in long-term psychiatry. Churchill Livingstone, Edinburgh
Wing J K, Morris B (eds) 1981 Handbook of psychiatric rehabilitation. Oxford University Press, Oxford

---

ADAPTATION

Adaptation is less well defined than the other processes in this section. As we have seen, it tends to get entangled with them, but it is nevertheless a most important and influential process in the context of occupational therapy.

In OT texts there are four distinct areas in which adaptation is discussed:

• **individual adaptation**, a combination of physiological, perceptual and cognitive responses to the environment

• **adaptive acquisition of skills, roles and occupations**
• **adaptations to occupations** in order to facilitate performance
• **adaptations to the environment** to promote access and facilitate performance.

Of these, individual adaptation is the most important aspect. If the individual cannot adapt, learning new skills may be seen as irrelevant and alterations to tasks or environments are unlikely to be seen as useful or beneficial and are likely to be rejected.

Individual adaptation

Individual adaptation tends to focus on the relationship between what the environment demands and what the person does to meet those demands. The individual is seen as adapting when the person is able to organize data and make a response that meets the demands (Reed & Sanderson 1992).

Adaptation is essentially 'an active process of engaging the environment according to one's intentions' (Kielhofner 1992). It involves the person in exercising perceptual discrimination, and cognitive and sensorimotor control.

Adaptation is the active use of personal potential and learning opportunities in order to reach personal goals and to exert influence on the environment. Development, in a purely biological sense, is a finite process which is largely predetermined and ends when maturation is completed, but adaptation, like learning, can and should continue throughout an individual's lifetime.

One may fail to adapt because of faulty learning, but one may also learn a behaviour which is maladaptive, such as stealing, or abusing drugs or alcohol. Seriously maladaptive behaviour is frequently associated with poor perceptions of personal control—the person either experiences his life as being controlled by others or by external circumstances, or he may seek to exert and impose personal control in maladaptive ways— through anger, bullying, abuse of another, or by 'antisocial' acts.

Humans are social beings who need to coexist with others within the boundaries accepted by a particular culture. Behaviour which is adaptive contributes to the individual's survival and well-being and to that of the society in which he lives. When an individual is adaptive he 'learns by his mistakes' but then uses that learning in order to predict and avoid similar mistakes in future. Behaviour which is maladaptive often fails to be predictive and either fails to meet the demands of the situation or actually makes the situation worse for the individual or someone else.

Adaptive behaviour should not, however, be equated with 'normal' behaviour (whatever that may be!), for slavishly following some perception of 'the norm', whether personal or cultural, may itself be maladaptive if what is required is change. Equally, behaviour which is idiosyncratic or even eccentric may sometimes be quite adaptive for the individual, even if society does not 'approve'.

Adaptive acquisition of skills

Mosey describes a developmental frame of reference which she calls 'recapitulation of ontogenesis' (ontogenesis means change over time, therefore Mosey means 'repeating stages of development'). She goes on to describe this as being:

addressed to the development of adaptive skills ... The term adaptive is used in the sense of being able to negotiate within the environment in such a way as to be able to satisfy one's own needs as well as those of others. It is used in the sense of creative use of the environment—not in the sense of conformity.

She lists six adaptive skills (see page 127) (Mosey 1986).

An adaptive continuum has been proposed, starting with basic physiological homeostatic reactions, developing in turn adaptive responses (motor, sensory, cognitive, intrapersonal and interpersonal), adaptive skills and adaptive patterns (Reed 1984, adapted from Kleinman and Buckley 1982).

Kielhofner includes adaptation as an occupational performance skill, the components of which are: notices/responds (reacts to environment); accommodates (modifies actions or location of available objects); adjusts (makes some change to environment, introducing a new element); benefits ('anticipates and prevents undesirable circumstances from recurring or persisting') (Kielhofner 1995).

Enabling a person to adapt is a matter of finding a balance between the demands of the environment and the needs, wishes and abilities of the person. People may be inhibited from adapting because the environment is unsuitable or because they do not have the right skills or information. They may be inhibited by their attitudes, motivation, thoughts and feelings. People who do not perceive or interpret the environment correctly—because of physical, cognitive or psychological deficits—find it difficult to adapt because they cannot modify their responses appropriately.

Adaptation to occupations

As the individual moves from childhood through adult life to old age, it is necessary for him to be able to adapt and change the pattern of roles, occupations and activities at each stage. What is appropriate in childhood is usually not socially acceptable in adult life; the vigorous young adult requires a different pattern of engagement from that of the older person. New social roles—student, parent, pensioner—bring with them the need for different patterns to be developed.

Many people manage this process of adaptation naturally and without problems, but others find the changes difficult, especially at significant points such as adolescence, or retirement, or when coping with stressful life events—marriage, separation, childbirth, bereavement, loss of job or ill health.

People may need assistance to adapt what they do in a number of ways. Changes can be made to the pattern and balance of occupations, to the nature of the activity, its sequence, complexity or duration, or to the tools and materials used.

Psychological or cognitive changes relating to occupations and activities may be even more important, for example moving from negative to more positive attitudes and patterns of thought, having expectations of success (or realistic judgement concerning likely failure), and setting achievable personal goals.

Successful participation in a variety of activities is seen as a means of promoting adaptation; the person may adapt by learning new skills, developing confidence and positive self-concept, and thus see himself as a competent performer who is capable of exercising a degree of control over his life.

Adaptation to the environment

The social environment may need changing so that people with whom the individual is connected give appropriate emotional support, cues or feedback to promote adaptive behaviour, or provide practical help.

Changing the physical environment, as in helping a disabled person to choose home adaptations and arranging installation of these is an important role for the therapist.

More subtle changes to the environment in terms of the level of stimulation and feedback it provides are also important in therapy and in certain learning situations.

Summary of the adaptation process

Metamodel: Organismic, emphasizing person–environment interactions and the necessity of continued personal change.

Origin of the problem: Problems of maladaptation may be due to developmental problems in basic perceptual and spatiotemporal adjustments in childhood, to maladaptive learning, to lack of suitable learning opportunities, to physical, cognitive, psychological or psychiatric problems which limit the ability to perceive and respond to the environment, to failure to cope with stressful life events, to inappropriate patterns of engagement in occupations and activities, to rigid or redundant routines and habits, or to barriers in the social or physical environment.

Primary assumptions
- The ability to react adaptively to changing circumstances throughout life is essential for personal survival and well-being.
- Adaptation depends on the ability to perceive and respond to stimuli in the environment and to learn new responses when required.
- A person may be enabled to respond more adaptively by enhancing perceptual skills and interpretive ability, providing feedback for responses, promoting successful engagement in relevant occupations, developing problem solving and planning skills, adapting tasks and environments to enhance performance.

Terminology: Adaptation; maladaptation; adaptive responses; adaptation factors.
Patient/therapist relationship: Most adaptative approaches are more or less client centred rather

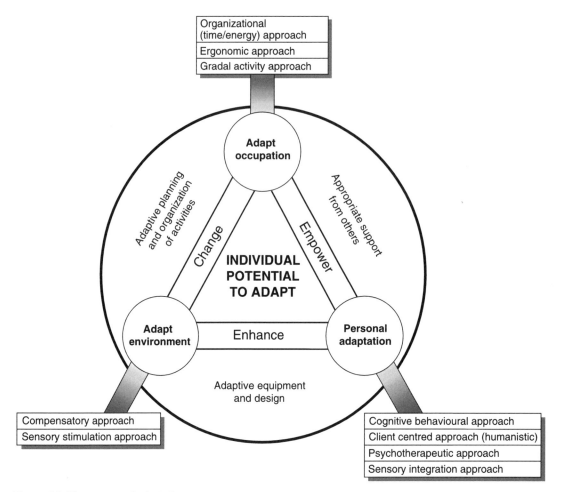

Figure 9.4 The process of adaptation.

than directive since taking control and making choices is seen as part of adaptive behaviour.

Application: Widely applicable in all situations and at all ages, providing age-appropriate techniques are selected.

Associated approaches: Adaptation through occupation (Reed and Sanderson 1992) (see p. 119); model of human occupation (Keilhofner) (see p. 114); adaptive skills (Mosey) (see p. 127); occupational adaptation (Schkade and Schultz 1994); adaptive response (King and Kleinman and Buckley: see Reed 1984); spatiotemporal adaptation approach (Keilhofner 1992); sensory integration approach (Ayres; King); sensory stimulation approach; cognitive behavioural approach; client centred approach; compensatory approach; organizational approach (energy conservation etc.).

Techniques: Various, as associated with above approaches; emphasis on teaching skills and facilitating responses to the environment, making appropriate environmental changes.

Criteria for evaluation of outcome: The person is able to respond adaptively to the situations which confront her; well-being is enhanced; survival is promoted; the individual is able to function within socially accepted norms.

Advantages: Expresses many of the fundamental concepts and principles of occupational therapy and provides a practical framework for interventions which include the person, his occupations and environment.

Disadvantages: The theory base is diffuse and not well presented. Much is based on hypotheses and assumptions which need further research.

Tends to make the assumption that an individual can always adapt, given the right assistance/environment, and does not take account of what to do when the individual appears incapable of change.

SUGGESTED READING

Personal adaptation

OT models which are based on adaptation are included in Section 4, with relevant texts.

see also:

Hopkins H, Smith H (eds) Willard and Spackman's occupational therapy, 8th edn. Lippincott, Philadelphia.

Ch. 4: section 3KD, Occupational adaptation (Schkade and Schultz). Ch. 9: 5B Assistive and adaptive Equipment. 5C Environmental adaptation.
Hagedorn R 1995 Occupational therapy perspectives and processes. Churchill Livingstone, Edinburgh. *Ch. 14: Occupational analysis and adaptation. Ch. 15: Environmental analysis and adaptation.*

> **Q** These four processes are widely used cross the whole spectrum of OT practice. Probably you use one or more yourself, or have seen them in use. With a colleague, or in a small group, discuss the following questions using your own experience to provide illustrations.
>
> 1 Why is it useful to distinguish between the four processes?
> 2 From your current case load, select a patient whose main problem seems to fit one of the processes. How are you treating this person and how did you decide which approaches/techniques to use?
> 3 Would a different process give a new perspective on this person and his/her needs?
> 4 Do therapists make good use of educational theory? Explore some applications of different leaning or teaching theories within your own practice.

THE PROBLEM BASED PROCESS MODEL

The problem based process model is a description of a process rather than a set of theories. It is derived from a personal model of practice which provides a means of using the occupational therapy process to integrate intervention using the processes of change which have previously been described. Although this model is not widely established, this description is included in the hope that it may assist therapists who prefer to take a process driven approach to their work to do so in a more structured and coherent manner, rather than being somewhat vaguely 'holistic' or 'eclectic'.

It is a person centred model, and the focus is on competent occupational performance in the areas of self-care, leisure and work (the individual may define these for himself). It aims to enable and empower the person to cope as well as possible, given individual circumstances, with the activities which he wants or needs to do, to a necessary or satisfactory standard, whenever required, and to experience optimum quality of life.

It is described as a problem based model because it seeks to use diagnostic reasoning to answer the question 'what is the problem?' by framing the problem situation in one or more of the following ways:

- **As a problem of development.** The person may have the potential to do more, but is unable to because he has not reached the developmental level necessary for functional performance. This may be because trauma has resulted in regression to a developmental level much lower than previously attained and not in balance with chronological age (e.g. following brain damage), or else that the person has for some reason (e.g.

genetic, environmental) never reached the necessary developmental level (is not yet able, can't yet do). Since skills cannot be learned until the individual is developmentally ready, therapy must be aimed at developing potentials for performance until the necessary level is attained.

• **As a problem of education.** The person may be developmentally ready and able to perform, but has never learnt how to do so, he lacks the necessary skill, knowledge, appropriate attitude or experience (would be able, doesn't know how to). Alternatively, new circumstances may require that new learning takes place. In either case, intervention needs to be aimed at helping the person to learn what is needed in order to function competently.

• **As a problem of rehabilitation.** The person was previously able to perform competently, but function has been lost as a result of illness or injury (was able, now can't do). In this case, therapy is aimed at restoring physical abilities or psychosocial skills to as near as possible to the previous level by a graded programme of activity.

• **As a problem of adaptation.** The person is confronted by a situation which cannot fundamentally be changed and to which he has failed to adapt (e.g. a permanent diasability or illness, a deteriorating condition, a set of challenging circumstances). In order to lead as full and satisfying a life as possible, adaptation must take place. Adaptation may be required to the environment, both social and physical, to the roles, occupations, activities and tasks which the individual wants and needs to perform, and to aspects of the individual himself — his attitudes, values, thoughts, emotions or skills.

The problem based process model is integrative, coordinating the use of compatible treatment approaches and techniques. Each process is complementary to the others, it is possible to change the emphasis from one process to another during different parts of the intervention, and to combine approaches from more than one process.

The use of this model represents a conscious attempt to view the person and his or her problems holistically and objectively before deciding on the nature of the problem and how (or if) to treat it. It places the person at the centre of this process and involves him closely in identifying and prioritizing problems in so far as this is possible for him.

Because the model is related to the problem and not to a particular frame of reference, a wide range of relevant treatment techniques or approaches can be synthesized providing that techniques do not clash. It avoids the lack of focus which can arise if techniques are used ecletically in the absence of a coordinating model of practice, and also the danger of taking too narrow a view. Because it involves processes which are well understood by others, it is highly suitable for use in a multidisciplinary setting.

Use of this model can be adapted to most locations and specialities, although it is of especial use where a variety of types of problems are seen, for example, in the community.

It can be used with an adaptation of the SOAP system, described in Chapter 2, in which the assessment phase involves identification of which of the four elements of the model best describes the problem.

Summary of the problem based process model

Metamodel: Pragmatic: it depends on the solution required by the problem.

Origin of the problem: No initial assumptions are made. The problem has first to be named, and then framed as one of Development, Education, Rehabilitation or Adaptation. This may lead to an explanation, or to one or more solutions for evaluation, and will suggest priorities. The nature of the problem is the key to subsequent action and choice of techniques or approaches.

Primary assumptions
• Performance problems can be analysed as being ones of development, education, rehabilitation or adaptation.
• Adequate data collection is essential for correct analysis of the problem.

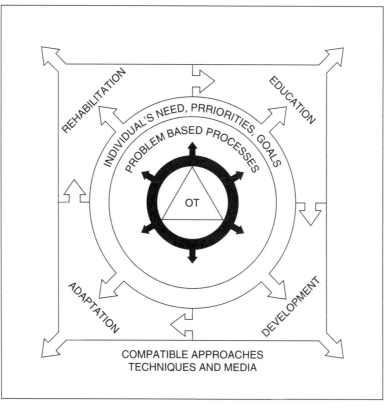

Figure 9.5 The problem based process model.

- The individual's perceptions of his problem are central to the process of analysis.
- The apparent problem may not be the real one: the apparent solution may not be the best one. Some problems do not have 'solutions', but all problems respond to action within an appropriate process of change.
- In any problem situation there may be several applicable solutions — one should keep an open mind.
- Interventions should be goal directed; goals must be negotiated by patient and therapist and defined before intervention begins.
- Progress should be monitored and action changed or the problem reassessed if results are ineffective.

Terminology: Processes of change; development; education; rehabilitation; adaptation; patient; client; therapist; occupational compe- tence; skill; problem based process; goal plan- ning; SOAP.

Patient/therapist relationship: Whenever possible the process is negotiated: the therapist assists the client to describe the problem and propose and evaluate solutions. The subsequent role of the client depends on the selected treatment approach.

Examples of Applications: Suitable for all types of patients/clients, particularly where complex situations/conditions are involved. Least suited to very straightforward cases where both prob- lem and solution are instantly obvious within a clear applied frame of reference.

Treatment techniques/approaches: Anything relevant to the problem (see those listed under each process), providing mutually incompatible techniques are not used simultaneously.

Criteria for evaluation of outcome: The previ- ously identified objective has been achieved and the identified problem is resolved.

Advantages: Highly pragmatic, flexible, avoids blinkered thinking. Suitable for all types of patients and can manage deteriorating or complex situations effectively. Promotes teamwork and provides measurable outcomes. Structured recording systems aid communication and evaluation.

Disadvantages: There may be too much focus on negatives, strengths and assets may be ignored. The whole system relies on very accurate assessment and identification of the problem, and correct framing of it within one or more of the four processes of change. Incorrect evaluation, wrong priorities or poor solutions render intervention inappropriate or ineffective. It is not a uniquely OT model, and may therefore lose its focus on occupational performance unless the therapist consciously maintains this. If the person centred focus is lost it may become overly reductive or directive.

10

Occupational therapy models

I have described the concept which underlies the creation of OT models as 'pure OT'. Of course, there is no such thing, for all knowledge comes from somewhere. But an OT model is one which presents theories which have been heavily filtered through an OT 'lens' together with ideas and techniques which are primarily derived from the practice of OT itself.

The models selected for description in this section are all based on views of the central importance of occupations in the life of the individual and their consequent value as therapy. They are mainly person centred and based on the processes of change discussed in Section 2, especially those concerned with the adaptive nature of human performance and the skills which people need in order to engage in occupations. Each author seeks to provide an integrated model to direct therapy, a guide to the application of techniques, and a means of distinguishing the unique contribution of OT from that of other professions.

It is important to read the most recent presentation of a model because these are developing entities, subject to change. A model which has ceased to evolve or to be discussed and analysed is very probably out of date. For this reason suggested reading tends to be restricted to the most recent texts. Earlier presentations of a model are of academic interest, and may help to show how it evolved and what the originators thought, but such 'history' can be confusing for the new student, whose chief need is to understand how a model is currently conceptualized and practised.

THE MODEL OF HUMAN OCCUPATION

The model of human occupation was first published in the *American Journal of Occupational Therapy* by Gary Kielhofner in collaboration with others (Kielhofner & Burke 1980; Kielhofner 1980a, b; Kielhofner & Igi 1980). He started the conceptualization which led to the model in the mid 1970s. These ideas have been developed in his book about the model (Kielhofner 1985) and he has continued to refine them over the past 15 years. In some respects his ideas have, therefore, changed. Kielhofner himself proposed his model as a basis for discussion and development, rather than as a complete and final explanation of OT practice.

In the 1985 presentation of the model Kielhofner views a person as an open system interacting with the environment and continually modifying it and being modified by it. The system is arranged as an hierarchy, composed of subsystems: volition (will); habituation (roles; rules); performance (skill). It focuses on the occupational areas of work, leisure and self-care. These fundamental elements of the model are mainly intact and are expanded in the 1995 version.

Although this model has generated a great deal of interest in the UK since the early 1980s, it should be remembered that it is only one of a large number of models in use in the USA, and not without its critics. The model has, however, been seminal and has provoked a much greater interest in model building and professional philosophy than existed previously in the UK.

This model may at first sight seem somewhat obscure due to the unfamiliar language and the detailed complexity of its structure. Once 'translated' the concepts become more familiar.

The model is an attempt at conceptualizing the underlying dynamics of human behaviour in terms of systems theory. An event anywhere in the system affects the whole system — 'resonates' through it — one must therefore consider the system as an indivisible, interrelated whole, and not attempt to reduce it to its parts. The elements of the system combine to produce (or fail to pro-duce) effective occupational behaviour. Each subsystem contains subsections. One significant recent change is that Kielhofner does not now view the system as hierarchical. In view of the very detailed presentation of systems theory and other important concepts, it really is essential to read the text to gain a complete understanding of the model; it is not possible to do more than present 'headlines' in this summary. Any attempt at summarizing the model in a few pages risks being reductionist — which is very much out of keeping with the scope and philosophy of the model.

Origins of the model

Kielhofner has drawn together a number of different areas of knowledge and a basic familiarity with these theories and their terminology is helpful. These include systems theory, cognitive psychology, developmental psychology, humanistic psychology and social psychology (including the theory of symbolic interactionism). Of these systems, theory is of fundamental importance, and a summary of this will be given shortly.

The 'OT roots' of the model stem from Mary Reilly, a respected American OT theorist whose work during the 1960s and 1970s has been highly influential. Reilly developed a hypothesis expressing the central belief of occupational therapy as follows: 'that man, through the use of his hands as they are energized by mind and will, can influence the state of his own health' (Miller & Walker 1993).

She developed the paradigm (or model) of occupational behaviour based on four concepts: 'the human need to be competent and to achieve; the developmental aspects of work and play; the nature of occupational role; the relationship of health and human adaptation' (Miller & Walker 1993), and went on to develop the concept of a work–play continuum and devoted much time to the study of the importance of play in human life. Reilly also became interested in open systems theory whilst developing her ideas.

Kielhofner was one of Reilly's students, he thought very highly of her, and his thinking has clearly been strongly influenced by her work.

The human open system

Kielhofner summarizes the main idea behind open systems theory as follows:

living phenomena are dynamic self-organizing entities exhibiting ongoing interaction with their environments (unless stated otherwise quotations are taken from Kielhofner 1995).

The dynamic aspect of this theory relates to flows of energy within the system; when new energy reaches a kind of critical mass, 'whole new states of organization emerge spontaneously'. He also states that 'components of a dynamical system behave in ways that cannot be predicted by their individual properties'.

The concepts of energy and organization are important. Because the human being is an open system, behaviour is influenced by the interactions of the human system, the task and the environment, and by the information which the environment and the task contribute to the situation. Kielhofner describes this as 'the "ballet" of ordinary occupational behaviour'. Behaviour is fluid and improvisational, 'spontaneously organized in real time and in the context of action'.

Kielhofner's ideas about the ways in which the human system is able to change adaptively include the following concepts:

- That new behaviour becomes established by repetition—by continually acting as a musician, or cook or football player the person gradually *becomes* it. Equally, if such behaviour is discontinued, the associated roles and skills also fade.
- That change can be produced by alterations within the organization of the internal system, or by changes external to it.
- That change can sometimes be dramatic and produces a whole new organization in a short space of time.
- Sometimes a small change in some significant factor can be the key to large changes in behaviour.
- The human system continually changes and adapts: 'the organization at any point in time is a reflection of the dynamic process of life'.

The internal organization of the human system

An open system operates by a process of circularity into, through and out of it.

Output, or the product of the system, is *occupational behaviour* which is classified as *work*, *daily living tasks*, *leisure* or *play*. Output is either adaptive or maladaptive (functional or dysfunctional).

Input (intake) to the system comes from the environment; it includes information from the surrounding people, events and objects.

Throughput processes input, organizes information, makes predictions on which to base action, and decisions on further action or output.

Feedback returns information to the system about the performance and consequences of action both from input and from monitoring of internal processes, e.g. how one feels about what one has done.

The three subsystems can be summarized as:

Volitional subsystem = Will. The mechanisms whereby we choose what to do.

Habituation subsystem = Roles and rules. The basic cognitive structures with which we organize our lives.

Mind-body-brain performance subsystem = Skills. The means by which we carry out occupational behaviour.

Subsystems of the model of human occupation

Volitional subsystem

'System of dispositions and self-knowledge that predisposes and enables persons to anticipate, choose, experience and interpret occupational behaviour.'

Volitional structure: 'Stable pattern of dispositions (cognitive/emotive orientations towards occupations) and self-knowledge (awareness of self as actor in the world) generated from and sustained by experience.'

Three areas of volitional structure:
- Personal causation (knowledge of capacity:

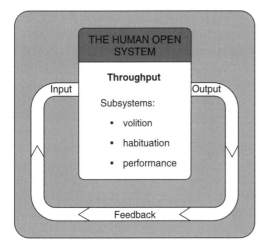

Figure 10.1 The model of human occupation. (Reproduced with permission from Creek J 1990 Occupational Therapy and Mental Health. Churchill Livingstone, Edinburgh.)

awareness of abilities; sense of efficacy: perception of control)
- Values (personal convictions; sense of obligation)
- Interests (attraction: enjoying certain activities; preference: enjoying certain ways of doing things).

Volitional process:

- Attending (attention; anticipation; reacting to possibilities)
- Experiencing (finding occupations enjoyable; feeling more or less able)
- Choosing (occupational and activity choices).

Volitional narratives: This is based on the ideas of Mattingly concerning the role of personal 'story-telling' as used by people to make sense of their lives (see narrative reasoning).

Habituation subsystem

'An internal organization of information that disposes the system to exhibit recurrent patterns of behaviour.' The operation of the habituation system involves processes and systems described in cognitive psychology.

Habituation structure:
- Habit (acquired by repetitions; operates at a

preconscious level to influence behaviour; habits involve cognitive processes)
- Habit map (guides the perception of familiar events and related action)
- Internalized roles (awareness of social identity with related obligations, situations and behaviour)
- Role scripts (understanding of social situations and expected responses)
- Influence of habits on occupational behaviour
- Influence of roles on occupational behaviour.

Habituation process: The organization of the subsystem guides immediate responses and also change over time. Principles include:

- Habit formation and change (habits: preserve patterns of behaviour; resist change; may outlive their usefulness)
- Socialization and role change (formal and informal roles change and need to be renegotiated throughout life).

The mind-brain-body performance subsystem

'Refers to the organization of physical and mental constituents which together make up the capacity for occupational performance.'

Constituents of the performance subsystem:
- Musculoskeletal system
- Neurological system
- Cardiopulmonary system
- Symbolic images (guide the system in producing behaviour).

The components of the subsystem receive, organize and process information in order to plan action and effect performance.

Kielhofner discusses the above subsystems at some length, and also explores environmental influences on occupational behaviour and the development of occupation. Occupational dysfunction is defined and explored within the terms and concepts of the model, together with methods for gathering data and the principles of therapeutic intervention. Considerable work on application has been carried out in the past 10 years and since this discussion is detailed and can only be appreciated in the original text, where case examples are given, no attempt will be made to summarize it here.

Much work has also been done to develop assessment tools for use within the model. These include the Occupational Case Analysis Interview (OCAIRS: Kaplan & Kielhofner 1989) and various checklists for role participation, personal interests, and self-rating of strengths and weaknesses (examples and cases are given in Kielhofner 1995).

One development resulting from the model has been research into skill in occupational performance. The taxonomy of skills is summarized in Table 10.1. Each skill has an associated list of actions.

This research into skills has resulted in the production of a detailed assessment instrument, the assessment of motor and process skills (AMPS). The assessment depends on very precise observations of the use of the listed actions in the context of functional performance. In order to use this, the therapist requires special training to become an accredited user. Development and research continue and this work may well have implications for use beyond the confines of the model of human occupation.

The influence of environment

Kielhofner stresses the importance of the effect of the environment on the individual. He describes 'press'—the demands which an environment places on an individual for appropriate occupational behaviours. The environment contains things which are capable of arousing us and promoting action—objects, tasks, social groups, cultural pressures—a degree of novelty and stimulation is pleasurable and promotes exploration and mastery. People generally perform well in such conditions.

Too much press, e.g. excessive novelty, over-stimulation, and being bombarded by the demands of an environment, results in stress, anxiety, uncertainty, helplessness, frustration, anger, overarousal and inability to cope (flight or fight responses). People fail to perform in such environments. Too little press results in apathy, withdrawal and disinterest, in which circumstances people also fail to perform well.

A continuum of function and dysfunction

In his earlier publications Kielhofner described a continuum stretching from expert function to total dysfunction. Functional occupational behaviour is achieved through *exploration* ('curious investigation in a safe environment to discover potentials for action and properties of the environment') which leads to *competence* ('striving to be adequate to the demands of a situation') and *achievement* ('striving to maintain and enhance standards of performance').

Dysfunction runs from *inefficiency* ('reduction or interference with performance resulting in dissatisfaction') to *incompetence* ('inability to routinely and adequately perform') and finally *helplessness* ('total or near-total disruption of performance').

In restoring function the patient may need to be taken through the stages of safe exploration until competence is achieved, and will then

Table 10.1 Motor and process skills

Motor skills	Process skills	Communication/ interaction skills	Social interaction skills
Posture	Energy	Physicality	Acknowledging
Mobility	Knowledge	Language	Sending
Coordination	Temporal organization	Relationships	Timing
			Coordinating
Strength and effect	Organizing space and objects	Information exchange	
Energy	Adaptation		

Adapted from Kielhofner (1995)

need to experience competent behaviour over a period of time in order to gain a sense of achievement.

Levy (in Willard and Spackman 1993) restates this idea in her description of 'the model of human occupation frame of reference'. However, in his most recent publication (1995), Kielhofner seems to have moved away from this concept, restricting himself to describing dysfunction within the terms of the model.

Putting the model into practice

I interpret the basic treatment principles of the model as asking a sequence of questions, and then directing interventions towards solving the perceived problems.

Volition

1 What does the patient most want, and why does she want it?
2 How does the patient perceive control in her life?
3 What does she like to do, and what is the pattern of her occupations — is this balanced?
4 Does she believe she is skilled and able to achieve?

Habituation

5 What roles has she had, does she have and will she perform?
6 What roles does she perceive herself as owning, and what obligations does she believe these place on her?
7 How well organized is her use of time?
8 Does she have adaptive, acceptable habits?
9 Is she rigid or flexible and able to adapt?

Performance

10 How skilled is she in all aspects of work, leisure and self-care?
11 What is her level of motor, process and social functioning in relation to occupations?
12 Are there any skills deficits?

(This list is, coincidentally, quite similar to that used in the OCAIRS.)

Summary of the model of human occupation

Metamodel: Organismic.
Origin of problem: Described within the language of the model as a dysfunction in volition, habituation or mind-body-brain performance.

Primary assumptions
- The human organism can be described as an open system.
- Occupations are central to human experience, survival and satisfaction.
- Occupational areas of work, self-care and play (leisure) evolve and change throughout the individual's life.
- Occupational performance results from the interaction of a dynamic system composed of volition, habituation and performance.
- People seek to explore and master their environments. Environment affords opportunities and presses for performance.
- The individual's perceptions of feedback from the environment are crucial in directing further output of adaptive occupational performance.

Terminology: Patient/client; therapist; intervention/treatment; adaption/maladaption; function/dysfunction; specific terminology of model (see previous notes).
Patient/therapist relationship: Therapist assesses problem, proposes problem solving intervention; explains model and implications; patient cooperates, may direct.
Examples of Applications: There appears to be no restriction on application: the literature deals with both psychiatric and physical dysfunction and learning disorders, and covers all age groups. However, the model is perhaps least appropriate for straightforward physical cases where a biomechanical approach will suffice, and the use of the model would be time-consuming and unwieldly.

Examples of Approaches: The model is strongly based on the application of occupations. Within that framework anything drawn from an organismic approach may be used, particularly cognitive and developmentally based techniques.

Evaluation of outcome: The patient shows improvement in defined deficits affecting the volition, habituation or performance subsystems, resulting in increased competence and achievement in occupational behaviour.

Advantages: A coherent set of theories is presented to direct the sequence and priorities of interventions. Psychological aspects of physical dysfunction are recognized. The model is widely applicable to all types of patients and may be particularly useful for unravelling complex problems. Patient motivation is regarded as crucial. It makes strong links between the individual, tasks and environment. Standardized assessments are used.

Disadvantages: The model is founded on an unproven and as yet relatively unresearched hypothesis about the basis of human behaviour. The concepts and language are complex. If dealing with a simple problem use of the whole process may be unwieldly, a 'sledgehammer to crack a nut'. The assessment process is thorough, but lengthy; as a result a problem may be well identified but a full programme may be overly time-consuming to implement. Access to appropriate assessment instruments is required. The model is biased towards volitional explanations of dysfunction, rather than physiological ones. The assessment of skills is weak on sensory skills/deficits. Behavioural and analytical techniques are not compatible with the philosophy of the model.

SUGGESTED READING

Kielhofner G 1995 A model of human occupation. Theory and Application, 2nd edn. Williams and Wilkins, Baltimore
Levy L L Model of human occupation frame of reference. In: Hopkins H L, Smith H D (eds) 1993 Willard &

Spackman's occupational therapy, 8th edn. Lippincott, Philadelphia
Miller R J, Walker K F 1993 Perspectives on theory for the practice of occupational therapy. Aspen, Gaithersburg (Ch. 7 Gary Kielhofner).

ADAPTATION THROUGH OCCUPATION

This model, like Kielhofner's, has evolved over some 15 or more years, and similarly is based on Reilly's work on occupational performance. It was first presented in 1980 in *Concepts of Occupational Therapy* by Kathleen Reed and Sharon Sanderson. This account is based on the 3rd edition, which was published in 1992 with some material from a summary of the model presented by Reed (1984).

Unlike the model of human occupation, the model is process driven, but it shares with the model of human occupation a focus on occupations as fundamental to human existence and health. Reed and Sanderson use a version of the human occupations model which depicts the individual as possessing sensorimotor, cognitive and psychosocial (formerly intrapersonal and interpersonal) skills, engaging in productivity, leisure and self-maintenance, and aiming for adaptation to and with the environment (Fig. 10.2).

The model, like Mosey's, is based strongly on the processes of development, learning and adapting. Participation in occupations and alterations of the environment are both seen as powerful mechanisms for change. The approach has become increasingly client centred. It is problem based, and considers problems as being grouped in four areas: biological, psychological, social and occupational. Of these the occupational element is central; the other areas overlap, giving rise to biosocial, psychosocial and biopsychological aspects.

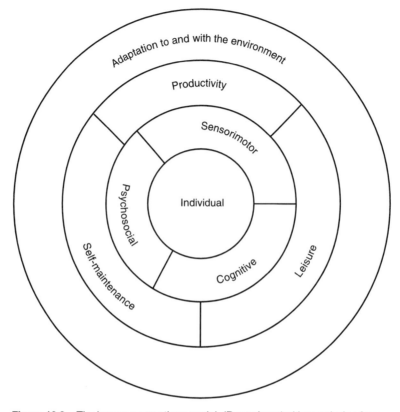

Figure 10.2 The human occupations model. (Reproduced with permission from Reed, Concepts of occupational therapy, copyright held by Wiliams & Wilkins, 1992.)

Reed and Sanderson are particularly concerned to identify the unique processes, concepts, techniques, concerns, assumptions and outcomes of OT. They focus on 'wellness', not the medical model which is concerned with 'illness'. Their view of the process and application of occupational therapy is highly structured. It is stressed that occupations can be therapeutic because they are the natural vehicles for normal development and adaptation and for the primary learning of skills. Skill assessment, development and retraining is seen as a main concern of occupational therapists. The OT can help the individual to develop adaptive responses through participation in occupations.

The key concepts of the model are discussed in detail and then expressed as a series of assumptions which underlie the practice of OT. Some of the key statements are summarized below.

Details of OT 'service programs', i.e. the services which OTs can provide in various specialties, are given, management aspects are explored, and there is a comprehensive glossary. This model is relatively accessible and has been quite widely adopted. It also forms the foundations for the development of the Canadian client centred model which will be described later.

Key assumptions

Assumptions about a human being

- **A person is**: a biopsychosocial and spiritual being; a unified whole; an open system energy unit; the sum total of the individual's life experience.

- **A person has**: the capacity for thought and sensation; needs; responsibilities; potential; basic rights.

Assumptions about occupational performance

These include statements concerning the central role of occupations in enabling the individual to continually change and adapt, meet responsibilities and change the environment, and the importance of occupations in maintaining health and a satisfying life. Occupations are determined by and occur in response to environmental factors.

Assumptions about occupational dysfunction

Dysfunction occurs when changes (ill health; injury; ageing; environment; etc.) affect the ability to use knowledge, skills or attitudes to adapt or adjust through the use of occupations.

Assumptions about health

Health is a total condition which is dynamic and changing. Illness affects occupational performance in several ways, including the reduction of energy, disruption of patterns and changing the person's abilities to perform occupations.

Assumptions about humanistic health care

These are philosophical statements concerning the person, the professional, the meaning of illness and the practice of health care which are difficult to summarize without losing their essence. The general thrust is optimistic and holistic, as expressed by the final statement 'both the person receiving care and the professional are whole human beings interacting in the healing effort.

Assumptions about receiving health care services

Statements of patient rights and expectations.

Assumptions about delivering health care through occupational therapy

These statements concern the aims of OT which should enable the client to:

- Achieve the highest level of occupational performance and adaptive behaviour consistent with the client's goal.
- Return to a normal living environment in the community if possible.
- Increase independent, adaptive behaviour and decrease dependent, maladaptive, or non-adaptive behaviour.
- Increase successful occupational performance and decrease non-productive occupational performance.

Health care programmes in occupational therapy are classified as:

- prevention
- developmental
- remedial
- environmental adjustment
- maintenance.

Assumptions about occupational therapy

The benefits of active doing in terms of promoting occupational performance and improving or restoring skills are described.

Therapy (in occupational therapy) is the use of directed, purposeful occupations to influence positively a person's sense of well-being and, thus, the state of a person's health.

Therapeutic occupations. These should be one or more of the following: meaningful; purposeful; goal directed; challenging. Reed offers an extended discussion of the individual and subjective nature of meaning in terms of occupational performance, and emphasizes the essentially purposeful nature of therapeutic activities (Reed 1984).

Assumptions about the therapeutic use of occupations

These statements summarize the rationale for the use of occupations as therapy.

The environment. Reed and Sanderson propose that occupational performance is influenced by the environmental context and content which may enhance or impede learning and performance. They suggest that analysis of the environment by the therapist is a significant therapeutic tool in identifying the causes of maladaptation and in enhancing and facilitating adaptive performance. The environment can be subdivided into:

- Physical environment: inanimate, non-human and natural aspects.
- Psychobiological environment: the individual self — the human being.
- Societal cultural environment: people and their cultures, attitudes, values and means of organization.

Occupations. These can be divided contextually into:

- self-maintenance
- productivity
- leisure

and into component *tasks* (but each occupation is performed as a gestalt).

Occupations have three *performance areas*. Each performance area requires the use of abilities and *skills* which are classified as:

- sensorimotor
- cognitive
- phychosocial
  - psychological (formerly intrapersonal)
  - social (formerly interpersonal).

Each of these skills is subdivided and defined.

The performance of occupations requires three *general elements* which are learnt:

- knowledge
- abilities
- attitudes/values.

In her 1984 summary of the model Reed also describes three *specific elements* related to occupational therapy:

- orientation: to time, place and person
- order: pattern and direction
- activation: ability to move and think.

Occupational adaptation and adjustment. The goal of the individual is life satisfaction through occupational adaptation. Occupations should enable the person to relate to the environment and to meet their needs by balanced performance within the areas of productivity, self-maintenence and leisure. Occupations have associated standards, roles and meaning for the individual. Occupational behaviour is either adaptive or mal/non-adaptive:

- Adaptive behaviour: uses skills to achieve balanced experience of occupations consistent with social norms and self-satisfaction.
- Maladaptive behaviour: is unsuccessful, and/or unacceptable to the individual or society.
- Non-adaptive behaviour: fails to produce an effective result, but is not unacceptable.
- Occupational dysfunction: problems in planning and/or performing an occupation; or in evaluating feedback of results.

Outcomes. In her 1984 summary of the model Reed states outcomes of occupational therapy clearly and concisely and these are best quoted as written:

- The person will be able to perform or have performed those occupations which meet the individual's needs and are acceptable to the person and society.
- The person will have the necessary performance skills which compose the occupations in the individual's repertoire of self-maintenance productivity and leisure.
- The person will have a balance of occupations such that actualization autonomy and achievement are attained to a maximum degree of adaptation.
- The person will be able to adapt to the environment or cause the environment to adapt to the individual.
- The person will be able to meet both deficiency needs and growth needs.
- Where the person is unable to perform skills independently, assistive devices or equipment or other environmental adjustments may be used. (Reed 1984)

Summary of adaptation through occupations

Metamodel: Organismic: humanistic/developmental/educational/adaptive.

Origin of problem: The patient shows dysfunctional, maladaptive, non-adaptive performance: the patient is unable to use a skill, does not use it, has not developed it, or never acquired it.

Primary assumptions

- A person changes, adapts, achieves satisfaction by means of occupational performance within physical and sociocultural environments.
- Occupational performance consists of learnt skills.
- Training in skills, engagement in occupations and/or modification of the environment can result in restoration of adaptive performance.

Terminology: Patient; therapist; therapy; function/dysfunction; adaptation/maladapation; description of environment; occupations; tasks; skills within terms of the model.

Patient/therapist relationship: A client centred, partnership model. The client's goals are used to direct the priorities of therapy.

Applications: Any person who, for whatever cause:

- has failed to develop occupational skills in any of the three areas
- who has temporary or permanent loss of occupational skills
- whose performance of occupational skills will require non-routine modification
- who is at risk for losing occupational skills. (Sanderson & Reed 1980).

Approaches: Any holistic approach appropriate to the problem. Cognitive-behavioural techniques may be appropriate, and neurodevelopmental and biomechanical ones are certainly suggested. Analytical techniques seem less relevant since they are not compatible with a strongly humanistic approach and the model does not pay much attention to unconscious mechanisms.

Advantages: A flexible, practical, holistic, client centred, problem solving approach; strong, coherent presentation of OT theory; compatible with a wide range of techniques. Focuses on 'wellness' not 'illness'.

Disadvantages: Few obvious ones: disregards unconscious motivations and says little about group processes which are not based on goal directed occupations. It is somewhat physically biased.

SUGGESTED READING

Reed K L, Sanderson S N 1992 Concepts of occupational therapy, 3rd edn. Williams and Wilkins, Baltimore

THE CANADIAN OCCUPATIONAL PERFORMANCE MODEL (GUIDELINES FOR CLIENT CENTRED PRACTICE)

The model evolved as a result of a joint initiative between the Canadian OT Association and the Canadian Department of National Health and Welfare (1983).

This began as an attempt to provide clear guidelines for practice, incorporating material which could be used to set standards and promote quality assurance. A principal objective was to develop an outcome measure for occupational therapy.

The task force produced reports which united a conceptual statement concerning the philosophy and principles of occupational therapy with practical guidelines for assessment and intervention, based on the OT process and using a client centred approach. Almost accidentally they also found themselves engaged in 'model making'.

The task group reviewed the available literature on OT theoretical and philosophical concepts, but the model has its main origins in Reed and Sanderson's presentation of the conceptual foundations of practice, and their view of occupational performance as consisting of a balance between work, leisure and self-care. Adaptation is viewed as 'a central unifying concept in the client centred practice of occupational therapy'. Activity is 'the core of the OT process' (CAOT 1991).

The model is shown in Figure 10.3. It should be compared with Figure 10.2 showing Reed and Sanderson's version.

The detailed report of the conceptual framework (Task Force Report 1983) deals with five elements:

• the worth of the individual
• holistic view of person
• occupational performance model

• therapeutic use of activity
• developmental perspective.

Law et al (1990) summarize the conceptual foundations of the model as a number of beliefs important to the practice of occupational therapy:

• that the individual client is an essential part of occupational therapy practice
• that the client should be treated in an holistic manner
• that activity analysis and adaptation may be used to effect change in the individual client's performance
• that an important consideration in the therapy process is the client's developmental stage
• that role expectations must be taken into consideration in assessing a client's performance. (Law et al 1990)

The model also describes (again following Reed) the importance of performance components (physical, mental, sociocultural and spiritual),

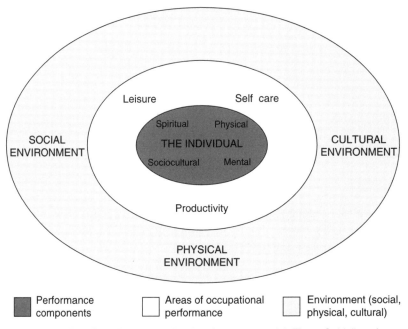

Figure 10.3 The Canadian occupational performance model. (From *Guidelines for the Client-Centred Practice of Occupational Therapy*, 1983. Reproduced with permission of the Minister of Supply and Services Canada, 1996.)

and of the environment (physical, social, cultural), and emphasizes the link between purposeful activity and health. Subsequent statements of the Guidelines (1986 and 1991) have refined the concepts and principles and the original conceptual model has now become a practice model (OT model).

As a conceptual model, the Canadian model of occupational performance now provides a useful statement of basic OT principles and philosophy together with a very clear presentation of the OT process. A distinguishing feature is the strongly client centred approach.

A critique of this model is given by McColl and Pranger (1994) who identify some inconsistencies and weaknesses in the connections between elements of the practice model, but agree that the conceptual model is useful.

Since Reed and Sanderson's model is now well developed and does make the links between practice and theory more explicit, it may be questioned why the Canadian task group felt that they had to create a new version. It is possible that they wished to simplify the rather densely argued original version, which is not always accessible to those not versed in theory.

However, whilst it lacks some of the evolved conceptualizations of similar models and does not completely explain the links between purposeful activity and improvements in health or occupational performance, it is very plainly an OT model. As the model has evolved (with influence from the model of human occupation), links between activities, skills, adaptation and mastery have been explored.

The occupational therapy process

The model is process driven; selection of approach is a consequence of assessment. The OT process is described by means of a systems approach. The associated flow chart illustrates the feedback links between stages more clearly than many of the linear models of the process, although the basic stages of the process are similar. Specific guidelines are given for implementation of each stage. This clarity makes this a useful means of communicating the essential practical

elements of OT practice to others, and provides OTs with a structure for audit and quality assurance, based on the structure – process – outcome formula developed by Donabedian (1980).

Key points are that programme planning must be based on an assessment of need, should indicate the specific plan for OT and how this links with other interventions, and, importantly, must involve the client in the preparation and implementation of the plan.

Goal planning

The client should, as far as is possible, determine her own priorities and set her own targets. Goals should be negotiated in relation to each unique individual and her situation. Goals relate to restoration, maintenance and development of function and to the prevention of dysfunction.

Selecting a frame of reference

A frame of reference is defined as 'a theoretical blueprint or a therapeutic philosophy within which programme planning may occur. The frame selected depends on the situation, resources, and the therapist's education and experiences' (CAOT 1991). In order to deal holistically with a client's needs, more than one frame of reference (approach) may be needed.

Intervention

Fundamental elements of intervention are described, including:

Spirituality. The need to try to understand 'the meaning of life' and also to make sense of one's self and one's experience as a human being is given importance. Therapists should offer clients the opportunity to explore existential themes such as suffering, guilt and forgiveness, joy, freedom or loneliness. The difficulty and sensitivity of this process is acknowledged.

Motivation. In OT motivation is linked with and achieved through the experience of participation in purposeful, meaningful, relevant daily activities.

The therapeutic relationship. 'A goal directed

interchange leading (the client) from constructive dependency to functional autonomy.' This is a personal and therapeutic relationship in which the following factors combine: the protagonists (therapist and client); foundations (mutual trust, non-judgemental concern and other attributes required by a client centred relationship—see pages 64 and 91); process of the relationship (starting; working; ending).

The teaching–learning process. Central in enabling the client to develop, change and adapt.

Ethics. Based on humanistic values.

Evaluation is described as essential. It is concerned both with audit of the effectiveness with which the stages in the OT process have been carried out and the achievement of the goals set at the start of treatment. Guidelines are given for this process.

Outcome measures

In their second report, *Towards Outcome Measures in Occupational Therapy* (1987), the task group gave an in-depth analysis of the problems and complexities of finding a satisfactory outcome measure. Law et al (1990) describe the development of the Canadian Occupational Performance Measure (COPM), and a summary is given in the manual (2nd edn 1994) which notes that 136 different outcome measures were researched, of which 54 were reviewed and criticized in relation to 10 criteria. Finding no instrument which was satisfactory or suitable for adaptation, the task group went on to design their own assessment.

The COPM is a criterion measure based on the client's own evaluation of her problems and priorities. The manual and assessment forms are now available in the UK (via COT) together with copies of the Guidelines (1991), or from the Canadian OT Association.

The assessment is simple to administer and score and requires practice, but no special training. It has five stages:

Problem definition. The client indicates the areas of self-care, productivity or leisure with which she is experiencing problems and rates these problems on a scale of 1–10 in terms of importance to her at present. If there are too many problems to tackle at once, those which seem less important at present are 'put on hold' until later in the intervention.

Problem weighting. The client is asked to use the 1–10 scoring system to indicate the degree to which she is able to perform each of the most important problem activities well, and her degree of satisfaction with performance.

The client's perceptions are accepted as valid without objective tests at this stage. If the client is unable to cope with this exercise a carer may do it for her, although, as the assessment is subjective, this is clearly less satisfactory.

Scoring. A simple calculation enables the therapist to give a rating to each activity as a baseline for intervention.

Goal planning can then be geared to the priority areas. COPM is seen as a first stage in goal setting, not as a replacement for other assessments, which may be needed to define the problem further once priorities have been set.

Reassessment. The assessment provides an outcome measure in terms of client scored improvement in performance and satisfaction once intervention is completed.

Follow-up. The client or care giver is asked if there are any further problems, in which case the assessment and intervention process is repeated.

This assessment is simple, fairly quick to use, can be used with a wide range of patients, and promotes a rapid identification of treatment priorities. It can specify problems across all performance areas. Problems which are not relevant or important to the client are not dealt with. The attention of both client and therapist is thereby focused on the problem solving process, and the relevance of therapy is explicit. Outcome measures are inbuilt.

The COPM is a versatile problem based assessment which can be used in a variety of settings, not necessarily in the context of the occupational performance model.

Summary of the Canadian occupational performance model

Metamodel: Holistic: the model takes a broad

view of the individual, and includes the spiritual aspect of experience. Developmental, educational and adaptive processes are important.

Origin of the problem: In general terms, problems are caused by an imbalance between the mental, physical, spiritual and social aspects of self leading to performance difficulties or deficits. This model pays less attention to defining the origins of dysfunction than to indicating courses of action to remedy it.

Primary assumptions: The holistic nature of the person requires holistic treatment; a client centred approach; need to consider individual roles, environment and experiences; the value of activities as therapy; the need to consider developmental level.

Terminology: Guidelines; client centred practice; occupational performance; dysfunction; adaptation; COPM.

Patient/therapist relationship: Strongly client centred; goals must be set by client.

Approaches: As required to deal with problems identified by client; must be activity based. Includes e.g. occupational performance; sensory integration; neurodevelopmental; behavioural; psychodynamic.

Examples of applications: Widely applicable; perhaps of less use when client is unable to participate in the goal planning process, although the carer may act as surrogate for the client.

Advantages: Strongly based on the OT process and occupational performance; involves the client at all stages; versatile, practical, accessible; avoids jargon; explains OT to others; provides standards and outcome measures.

Disadvantages: Practice model is still developing and may lack a degree of academic rigour and cohesion.

SUGGESTED READING

Canadian Association of Occupational Therapists (1991) Occupational therapy guidelines for client centred practice. CAOT Publications, Toronto
Law M et al 1990 The Canadian Occupational Performance Measure: an outcome measure for occupational therapy, CJOT 57 (2): 82–87

Law M et al 1992 Canadian Occupational Performance Measure (manual), 2nd edn. CAOT Publications, Toronto
McColl M A, Pranger T 1994 Theory and practice in the occupational therapy guidelines for client centred practice. CJOT 61 (5): 250–259

ADAPTIVE SKILLS

In contrast to the previous generic models, that proposed by Ann Cronin Mosey is primarily related to psychiatric practice. Her ideas were first developed during the late 1960s and early 1970s, but her important book *Psychosocial Components of Occupational Therapy* (1986) provides a synthesis of previous ideas. Like Reed, she views occupational therapy as being primarily concerned with skills and adaptation, and she has strong views about the legitimate tools and concerns of the profession. Like Kielhofner, she uses the systems language of input, throughput, output and feedback to describe the OT process. She does not herself describe her ideas as a 'model' since she reserves that term for the higher level which other writers

term a paradigm. In terms of organization and integration, however, it clearly compares with other models described in this section.

Her model deals with problems in psychosocial function. She explains these as either a learned maladaptive response, or a lack of skill affecting task planning and performance, interactions, or ability to identify and satisfy needs.

In this context she lists four *performance components*:

- sensory integration
- cognitive function
- psychological function
- social interaction.

These four components are used in five areas of *occupational performance*:

- family interactions
- activities of daily living
- school/work
- play/leisure/recreation
- temporal adaptation.

Occupational performance takes place in the context of the environment, which can be divided into *cultural environment, social environment* and *physical environment*.

Three frames of reference

These are proposed for use in psychiatric occupational therapy. All three frames of reference deal with the use of activities as vehicles for skill or role development.

The *analytical frame of reference* is described as being appropriate when dealing with a client whose life situation involves difficulties with 'universal issues'. These are listed as reality, trust, intimacy, adequacy, dependence/independence, sexuality, and aggression. Her interpretation of the analytical approach is eclectic, but appears to be based more on object relations theories than Freudian ones.

The *acquisitional frame of reference* has a cognitive/behavioural base, and deals mainly with the acquisition of interpersonal skills and roles.

In *recapitulation of ontogenesis* Mosey uses a developmental/humanist frame of reference, but links this with elements of cognitive and social learning theory. She identifies six (originally seven, drive-object skill was removed from later lists) *adaptive skills*. These skills are acquired sequentially and are universal. They include:

- Perceptual motor skill. The ability to receive, select, combine and coordinate vestibular, proprioceptive and tactile information for functional use.
- Cognitive skill. The ability to perceive, represent and organize sensory information for the purpose of thinking and problem solving.
- Dyadic interaction skill. The ability to participate in a variety of dyadic relationships.
- Group interaction skill. The ability to engage in a variety of primary groups.

- Self-identity skill. The ability to perceive the self as a relatively autonomous, holistic and acceptable person who has permanence and continuity over time.
- Sexual identity skill. The ability to perceive one's sexual nature as good and to participate in a relatively long-term sexual relationship that is oriented to the mutual satisfaction of sexual needs. (Mosey 1986: Note: this list is taken from her most recent publication, and differs in some small but significant aspects from her previous definitions.)

These adaptive skills are composed of *adaptive subskills* which in turn are composed of *skill components*. Perhaps the most interesting and potentially useful part of the model is the analysis of each of the six skills as a developmental sequence, linked to chronological developmental stages in which each skill evolves in complexity and adaptive potential. An assessment of the level of function therefore enables one to determine a developmental age or level for the individual in each skill. This enables activities and interactions to be selected at the correct level so that early skills can be learnt or regained before later ones and the correct developmental sequence is retained. (This is similar to the approach of Allen (1985), who proposes a cognitive/developmental system using very well structured activities aimed at identified levels, see page 131.)

Assessments and interventions are related to each of these areas, depending on the type of dysfunction, and a range of standardized tests is proposed.

In common with Reed and Kielhofner, Mosey quotes Reilly and emphasizes the use of activity, both for individuals and in structured groups. Experiential learning through activity, interactions and group work is seen as the means of producing adaptive responses or improving skills.

Like Reed, she is concerned with 'wellness' rather than 'illness' and suggests a list of 'health needs' which a therapist should be aware of and should attempt to meet through occupational therapy programmes. Because her base is in psychiatric practice, the purpose of this list seems largely to be to foster anti-institutionalized relationships and programmes.

This list has similarities with Maslow's hierarchy of needs, and includes:

- psychophysical needs (physiological, environmental)
- temporal balance and regularity (varied pattern of occupations and timing)
- safety (physical and emotional)
- love and acceptance (client / therapist relationship
- group association (sharing)
- mastery (successful participation in activity)
- esteem (a valued, rewarding role)
- sexual needs (recognizing needs; enabling needs to be met)
- pleasure (client's individual definition)
- Self-actualization (meaningful activities and relationships).

Mosey presents a detailed and densely argued account of occupational therapy which cannot be encapsulated in a few pages. Her ideas are pragmatic and those who find them interesting are recommended to try and obtain her book. (Mosey does not give a visual representation of her ideas, and it would be presumptuous to invent one.)

Summary of the adaptive skills model

Metamodel: Organismic. Reed (1984) criticizes the model as philosophically inconsistent because it combines deterministic elements from behaviourism and analytical theory with developmental / humanist theories. Whilst Mosey does discuss the three frames of reference, she does not imply simultaneous use, but rather sees these as alternatives, based on a pragmatic, problem solving approach to a client's needs. The model remains basically holistic.

Origin of problem: Lack of adaptive skills due to incorrect or incomplete learning; disrupted maturation or incomplete developmental sequence; environmental stress; physical or psychological abnormality.

Primary assumptions

- Adaptive skills are required for the satisfactory performance of activities and interactions.
- Adaptive skills are learnt, and can be trained or regained in a developmental sequence.
- Therapeutic activities and interventions should be pitched to match the initial developmental level of the individual and progressed as the individual masters each stage.

Terminology: Client / patient; therapist; therapy; adaptive skills; function / dysfunction; adaption / maladaption.

Patient/therapist relationship: Therapist assesses and provides prescribed intervention; patient cooperates and may assist with goal setting. The value of the development of a trusting, caring relationship between client and therapist, and the therapist's 'conscious use of self' as a therapeutic tool is emphasized.

Examples of applications: Psychiatric disorders, both acute and long term. People who have symptoms of psychosocial dysfunction.

Approaches: Analytical; acquisitional; developmental.

Examples of techniques: Those relevant to the selected approach. Within recapitulation of ontogenesis these are related to the six adaptive skills and may include: activities to promote sensory integration; cognitive activities; perceptual activities; dyadic and group interactions and activities; activities to enhance self-image and identity; sexual counselling and interactive role-play; behavioural learning techniques; social modelling.

Advantages: A flexible and non-dogmatic approach widely applicable in psychosocial dysfunction. Activity based. Recognizes that progress cannot be achieved if the individual has not reached the required developmental level — identifies level and assists correct choice of activity in correct sequence. Useful for individuals functioning at low level.

Disadvantages: The strongly psychosocial emphasis leads to restricted applicability in physical settings.

SUGGESTED READING

Mosey A C 1973 Activities therapy. Raven Press, New York
Mosey A C 1981 Occupational therapy, configuration of a
  profession. Raven Press, New York
Mosey A C 1986 Psychosocial components of occupational
  therapy. Raven Press, New York

Miller R J, Walker K F 1993 Perspectives on theory for the
  practice of occupational therapy. Aspen, Gaithersburg.
  Ch. 3: Anne Cronin Mosey

THE COGNITIVE DISABILITY MODEL

This model has been developed over the past 20 years in the USA by Claudia Allen, originally as an alternative model for the treatment of chronic psychiatric disorders, especially those resulting in impairments to the individual's ability to cope with basic daily tasks. It is a more limited model than others in this section, but it shares their focus on therapeutic activity.

Allen realized that the rehabilitation process, with its implied expectation of recovery, and the traditional focus on 'stretching abilities' as a means of achieving improvement, did not produce the expected results in patients with chronic disorders in which cognitive function was diminished or liable to decline.

Drawing on theories from cognitive, developmental and biological perspectives in psychology, this perception led her to challenge the applicability of the concepts on which traditional therapy was based. Her conclusions were considered radical when she first proposed them and are still viewed by some as controversial.

She developed the concept of 'cognitive disability': 'a restriction in voluntary motor action originating in the physical or chemical structures of the brain and producing observable limitations in routine task behaviour' (Allen 1985).

She hypothesized that a cognitive disability was due to actual brain damage, be it chemical (temporary or permanent) or anatomical. This damage reduced normal function. Six levels related to cognitive function could be observed and described.

Allen uses information processing models of cognition, and describes the following factors as contributing to task performance: attention to sensory cues; motor actions; conscious awareness; purpose; experience; process; time.

The crucial, and at the time controversial, part of her theory, was the view that an individual could only function within the limits of his/her cognitive level and could not be expected to function above this level unless some fundamental change occurred as a result of medication or the remission of illness. She created task related tests by means of which the level of cognitive function could be assessed.

Allen states her rationale quite boldly: 'Therapists might assume that a description of six levels will direct our services towards increasing the cognitive level. Implicit in the assumption is a question: can occupational therapy change the cognitive level? The answer is no, at least for the present' (Allen 1985).

She goes on to suggest that it is pointless to bewilder and frustrate individuals with cognitive disabilities by presenting them with challenging tasks or situations to which they are unable to respond. Instead, she proposes that tasks, tools, and environment need to be structured very precisely to compensate for deficits and produce optimum performance at each level.

Since this initial presentation of her theories, Allen has refined and evolved them, and they have been applied in fields other than psychiatry, for example the treatment of head injuries, CVE (strokes); learning disabilities, dementia, and other disorders where cognitive disability is a feature.

Task analysis and environmental analysis

At each level different forms of tasks, presentation of information, tools and materials, and arrangement of environmental cues are required. These are described in detail, and are of interest beyond the confines of the model, providing a clear example of the occupational therapist's approach to the therapeutic application and adaptation of activities.

Perhaps because the model was generated in the context of long-stay psychiatry, Allen has developed the use of simple craft projects typically employed in large institutions, both as illustrations of the necessary adaptations for each level, and also as a means of assessment.

Whilst some have welcomed this specific use of traditional crafts, therapists who are less drawn to the making of mosaic trivets and leather thonging have found this restricting, however, the general approach can readily be adapted for use with simple daily living tasks such as cooking.

Assessments

The Allen Cognitive Level (ACL) test uses performance at leather lacing (thonging) as a test of cognitive ability.

This task is too complex for some patients and the lower cognitive level test, which asks the patient to imitate the action of clapping, was designed for patients at levels 1, 2 or 3.

The routine task inventory (RTI) is a daily living checklist rated by interview and/or observation, with four subscales dealing with areas of work, communication, physical activity and communication.

These assessments are marketed in the UK together with a manual and use does not require special training.

Approach

The cognitive disabilities model mainly uses a compensatory approach, seeking to maximize residual function through task adaptation and environmental adaptation. The emphasis is on adapting the task and the circumstances of performance to match the abilities of the individual, rather than expecting the individual to change or adapt.

Allen locates the points at which change can be made in the life of an individual (structure;

| Box 10.2 | Six cognitive levels |

Level 1: Reflexive (automatic actions)
The individual seems unaware of external environment or stimuli. Only simple, single, automated, gross patterns of movement are initiated. No constructive tasks can be attempted; one word instructions may trigger an automatic response. Actions are not imitated if demonstrated.

Level 2: Movement (postural actions)
The individual attends to her own movement, or that of others, or of objects. Movement follows simple gross motor patterns, e.g. pacing, rocking, with no purpose except seeking comfort. Some actions may be imitated, but little or no purposeful task performance is achieved.

Level 3: Repetitive actions (manual actions)
Objects are the centre of attention, and are repetitively explored or manipulated, but with little purpose. Objects are recognized as separate from self, but the patient is unaware of others and is generally disorientated. Very simple repetitive actions may be attempted under close instruction and supervision but attention span is very short.

Level 4: End product (goal directed actions)
The individual is able to pay attention to the tangible elements of her environment as long as these are within view and reach. A thing out of sight 'disappears' and will not be looked for. A very familiar repetitive task can be completed, or a simple pattern or demonstration followed slowly, one step at a time, with verbal cues. Task completion brings satisfaction. Judgement is poor and problem solving virtually non-existent.

Level 5: Variations (exploratory actions)
Allen says that a percentage of the 'normal' population functions at this level. The individual is able to initiate actions to achieve personal goals, and can adjust actions as the task progresses to some extent, e.g. finding missing item but has trouble planning ahead, anticipating or solving problems except by trial and error. Personal needs come first, and the person does not usually think before she acts, or pause to consider the consequences.

Level 6: Tangible thought (planned actions)
The individual is capable of symbolic thought, uses reasoning and problem solving and is capable of showing initiative and creativity. Complex activities and chains of activities can be completed. Level 6 is associated with a higher educational and occupational background.

---

process; environment) and shows how the adaptive models, which expect the patient to make changes to meet new demands, are inappropriate for people who are unable to cope with new learning, and for whom a 'magical cure' is unlikely.

Research base

Research into this model has been quite extensive and continues.

Summary of the cognitive disability model

Metamodel: Reductionist.

Origin of the problem: Cognitive dysfunction due to chemical or physical changes in the brain, adversely affecting motor performance.

Primary assumptions
- Effective performance depends on intact cognition.
- OT cannot improve cognition if deficit is due to brain damage.
- When a cognitive disability is present, the therapist may help the patient to compensate for this by use of environmental cues and adaptations and by using task analysis.

Terminology: Cognitive disability; cognitive levels; task analysis; environmental adaptation.

Patient/therapist relationship: Therapist is supportive but directive.

Examples of applications: Chronic psychiatric conditions such as psychotic disorders; learning disabilities; brain damage;

Approaches: Cognitive disabilities (diagnostic); compensatory.

Advantages: Recognizes the reality that some people cannot change adaptively, have limited abilities, and require special help to maximize their residual skills. Has a simple set of diagnostic assessments. The concepts are coherent and well explained. The model removes the sense of professional frustration resulting from failure to achieve 'improvement'.

Disadvantages: It is possible that, in institutional settings, the reductive nature of the model may result in a patient becoming labelled as for example 'a level 3', and that this may negatively affect staff perceptions and result in self-fulfilling prophesies of low performance, and failure to recognize change due to chemotherapy or remission of illness (certainly not what the author intended). The model has a very narrow theoretical base and discounts other explanations for dysfunction, for example, motivational ones. The dogmatic statement that OT cannot improve cognition requires further research.

SUGGESTED READING

Allen C A 1985 Occupational therapy for psychiatric diseases; measurement and management of cognitive disabilities. Little Brown, Boston
Allen C A 1992 Cognitive disabilities. In N Katz (ed) Cognitive rehabilitation: Models for intervention in occupational therapy. Andover Medical Publishers, Boston
Kielhofner G 1992 Conceptual foundations of occupational therapy. F A Davis, Philadelphia

Levy L L 1993 Cognitive disability frame of reference. In: Willard and Spackman's Occupational Therapy. Lippincott, Philadelphia
Miller R J, Walker K F 1993 Perspectives on theory for the practice of occupational therapy. Aspen, Gaithersburg. *Ch. 8: Claudia Allen*

THE ACTIVITIES HEALTH MODEL

This model was originally developed by Simme Cynkin in the 1980s in the USA. It was later presented in a more evolved form (Cynkin and Robinson 1990) together with a student centred, experiential activities based curriculum for OT education.

Like most American models produced during this period, it owes a debt to Mary Reilly's work on occupational performance. It differs from other models in focusing on 'activities' rather than 'occupations' and describing participants as 'actors'. (The difference may be academic, but has possibly lost Cynkin some support for not using the terminology of occupational performance adopted by other American theorists.)

It is, perhaps, a little less well conceptualized

than some of the more tightly argued theoretical models, but its value lies in the authors' deep understanding of the subjective nature of engagement in activities, the importance of activities in the lives of individuals, and the link between activities and health. It is as much a statement of philosophy as it is of practice. Students are encouraged to undertake various tasks and reflect on these in order to understand the scope and meaning of their own experiences as actors.

The model adopts a strongly client centred approach, emphasizing the idiosyncratic nature of experience and the personal meanings and emotions which activities evoke.

It is not a model which is widely known or used in the UK and it is included in this section principally because it offers a provoking discussion of the richness of human participation in activities, and the ways in which the therapist can respond to this richness and use it as a means of therapy.

Assumptions about activities

Cynkin explores a number of assumptions which are keys to the concept of activities health. These are based on theories derived from behavioural, cognitive, educational and social psychology and sociology.

- Activities of many kinds are characteristic of and define a human existence.
- Activities are socioculturally regulated by a system of cultures, beliefs and customs and are thus defined by and in turn define acceptable norms of behaviour.
- Change in activities related behaviour can move in a direction from dysfunctional to functional.
- Change in activities related behaviour from dysfunctional to functional takes place through motor, cognitive and social learning. (Cynkin and Robinson 1990).

Challenges to occupational taxonomies

Cynkin criticizes the usual work/leisure/self-care division as too restrictive and points out that perception of role and the nature of participation is highly individual. Sociobiological and sociocultural classifications are proposed as alternatives.

Activities health

This is defined as follows:

a state of well-being in which the individual is able to carry out the activities of daily living with satisfaction and comfort, in patterns and configurations that reflect sociocultural norms and idiosyncratic variation in number, variety, balance and context of activities.

The activities health assessment

This involves highly detailed examination of the individual's *activities configuration*.

The patterns of engagement of the individual, the appropriateness and balance of these and the level of individual satisfaction and comfort are used as measures of activities health. Various self-rating assessments are used to explore these aspects and a detailed history of participation is obtained.

Occupational therapy and activities health

Activities, to foster health, require the following of the actor: the use of the hands; conscious problem solving; creative activity.

Cynkin explores the ways in which activities of daily living are 'both ends and means in the practice of occupational therapy'. Activities engage the actor in a very special way: by performing an activity you become increasingly the thing you are trying to be—taking on the roles, skills, culture, meanings of the activity. (A similar concept is also developed by Kielhofner (1995)). Therefore, through engagement in systematically selected activities, function can be developed and restored.

Activities analysis within this model includes far more than the usual 'skills based' format. It involves having an appreciation of the historical and cultural significance of each activity, and its subjective and phenomenological

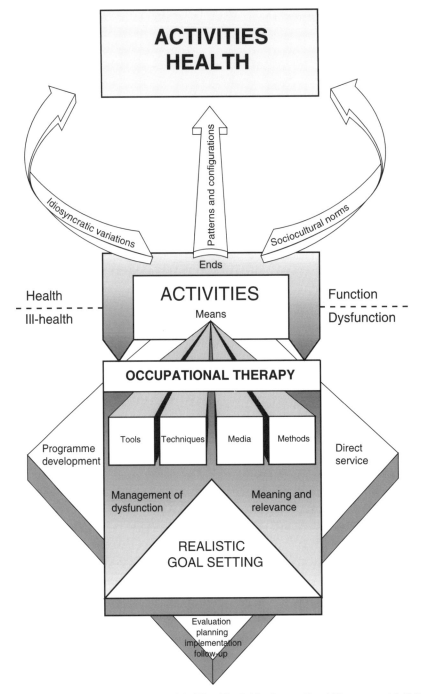

Figure 10.4 The activities for health model. (After Fig. 5.1 in *Occupational Therapy and Activities Health* by Cynkin, 1990, with permission. Published by Little Brown and Company.)

aspects—symbolism, personal meanings, personal preferences and style, feelings, effects of environment.

A version of the usual occupational therapy process is used to structure therapy.

Summary of the model of activities health

Metamodel: Holistic.

Origin of the problem: Activities health has been affected, as shown by assessments (various causes).

Primary assumptions: As summarized above: engagement in activities is equated with health; failure to engage signals ill-health or dysfunction.

Terminology: Activities health; dysfunction; function; activity analysis.

Patient/therapist relationship: A client centred partnership model.

Examples of applications: A wide selection of physical, developmental and psychiatric case studies are given implying widely applicable use with a wide age range.

Examples of approaches: Therapy must be activity based and the graded activities approach and educational approaches are predominant, however, these may be employed from biomechanical, neurodevelopmental, cognitive-behavioural, cognitive-perceptual or projective (psychotherapeutic) perspectives; the compensatory approach may be used. Little reference seems to be made of group work and analytical theories do not appear to have much place in this model.

Advantages: Places a great emphasis on the applied use of activities and on activity analysis; therapists educated in the philosophy and practice of this model are likely to have a deep appreciation of the subjective aspects of activities and their role in promoting health. The emphasis is on 1:1 treatment rather than groupwork.

Disadvantages: It is less clear (in the text) how these principles should be applied in practice: descriptions of therapy tend to be similar to those where other frames of reference are in use. The assessment seems likely to take more time than will be available in many treatment settings. The research base is unclear.

SUGGESTED READING

Cynkin S, Robinson A M 1990 Occupational therapy and activities health: towards health through activities. Little, Brown & Co., Boston

---

Bibliography

Abraham B 1988 The dilemmas of helping someone towards independence: an experiential account. British Journal of Occupational Therapy

Allen C K 1985 Occupational therapy for psychiatric disorders: measurement and management of cognitive disabilities. Little Brown, Boston

Allen 1992 Cognitive disabilities. In: Katz N (ed) Cognitive rehabilitation: models for intervention in occupational therapy. Andover Medical Publishers, Boston

American Association of Occupational Therapy 1995 Position Paper: occupation. AJOT 49(10): 1015–1018

American Association of Occupational Therapy 1995 The philosophical base of occupational therapy. AJOT 49(10): 1026

American Journal of Occupational Therapy 1991 45(11)

Arnold M E, Penn B 1990 Expert systems and occupational therapy. British Journal of Occupational Therapy 53(9): 365–368

Atkinson R L, Atkinson R G, Smith E, Benn D 1993 Introduction to psychology, 11th edn. Harcourt Brace Jovanovich, Florida

Baron R A, Byrne D 1987 Social psychology, 5th edn. Allyn and Bacon, Massachussetts

Balint M 1984 The basic fault. Arrowsmith, Bristol

Bandura A 1977a Social learning theory. Prentice Hall

Bandura A 1977b Self-efficacy: towards a unifying theory of behaviour change. Psychological Review 84: 191–215

Barnitt R 1990 Knowledge, skills and attitudes; what happened to thinking? British Journal of Occupational Therapy 53(11): 450–456

Barris R 1982 Environmental interactions, an extension of the model of human occupation. American Journal of Occupational Therapy 36 (10)

Benner P 1984 From novice to expert: excellence and power in clinical nursing practice. Maddison-Wesley, Massachusetts

Bigge M 1987 Learning theories for teachers, 4th edn. Harper & Row, New York

Bion W R 1961 Experience in groups. Tavistock Publications, London

Bobath B 1986 Adult hemiplegia: evaluation and treatment, 2nd edn. Heineman, London

Brewin C R 1988 Cognitive foundations of clinical psychology. Lawrence Erlbaum, Hove

Bruce M A, Borg B 1987 Frames of reference in psychiatric occupational therapy. Slack, New Jersey

Bruner J 1990 Acts of meaning. Harvard University Press, Cambridge, MA

Bumphrey E (ed) 1987 Occupational therapy in the community. Woodhead & Faulkner, Cambridge

Burke J P, DePoy E 1991 An emerging view of mastery excellence and leadership in occupational therapy practice. AJOT 45(1): 1027–1032

Canadian Association of Occupational Therapists 1991 Occupational therapy guidelines for client centred practice, CAOT, Ontario

College of Occupational Therapists 1994 Core skills and a conceptual foundation for practice: a position statement. COT, London

Creek J (ed) 1990 Occupational therapy and mental health: principles, skills and practice. Churchill Livingstone, Edinburgh

Creek J (ed) 1996 Occupational therapy and mental health: principles, skills and practice, 2nd edn. Churchill Livingstone, Edinburgh

Cynkin S, Robinson A M 1990 Occupational therapy and activities health: toward health through activities. Little Brown & Co, Boston.

Donabedian A 1980 The definition of quality and approaches to assessment. Health Administration Press, Michigan

Douglas T 1976 Groupwork in practice. Tavistock Publications, London

Drouet V M 1986 Individual behavioural programme planning with long-stay schizophrenic patients. British Journal of Occupational Therapy 49(7)

Dryden W, Golden W (eds) 1986 Cognitive behavioural approaches to psychotherapy. Harper and Row, London

Eagan G 1986 The skilled helper. Brooks Cole, California

Eggers O 1988 Occupational therapy in the rehabilitation of adult hemiplegia. Heineman, London

Finlay L 1988 Occupational therapy practice in psychiatry. Croom Helm, London

Fleming M H 1991 The therapist with the three-track mind AJOT 45(11): 1007–1014

Foulkes S H, Anthony E J 1965 Group psychotherapy: the analytical approach. Penguin, Harmondsworth

Gagné R M 1977 The conditions of learning and theory of instruction, 3rd edn. Holt Saunders

Galley P M, Forster A L 1987 Human movement, 2nd edn. Churchill Livingstone, Edinburgh

Gerard B A, Boniface W J, Howe B H 1980 Interpersonal skills for health professionals. Reston, Virginia

Goodwill C J, Chamberlain M A (eds) 1988 Rehabilitation of the physically disabled adult. Croom Helm, London

Grant L, Evans A 1994 Principles of behavioural analysis. Harper Collins College Publishers

Gross R 1992 Psychology: science of mind and behaviour, 2nd edn. Hodder and Stoughton, London

Hagedorn R 1995a Occupational therapy perspectives and processes. Churchill Livingstone, Edinburgh

Hagedorn R 1995b The first intervention: an exploratory study of clinical decision making in occupational therapy. MSc (unpublished), University of Exeter

Heap K 1979 Process and action in working with groups. Pergamon Press, Oxford

Hopkins H, Smith H (eds) 1993 Willard and Spackman's occupational therapy, 8th edn. Lippincott, Philadelphia

Howe M C, Schwartzberg S L 1986 A functional approach to group work in occupational therapy. Lippincott, Philadelphia

Hume C, Pullen M 1986 Rehabilitation in psychiatry. Churchill Livingstone, Edinburgh

Johnson-Laird P N, Wason P C 1977 (eds) Thinking: readings in cognitve science. Cambridge University Press, Cambridge

Javetz Katz 1989 Knowledgeability of theories of occupational therapy practitioners in Israel. American Journal of Occupational Therapy 43: 10

Jones M C 1983 Behaviour problems in handicapped children. Souvenir Press, London

Jones M 1960 An approach to occupational therapy. Butterworths, London

Jones M, Jay P (ed) 1977 An approach to occupational therapy, 3rd edn. Butterworths, London

Kaplan K, Kielhofner G 1989 Occupational case analysis interview and rating scale. Thorofare, N J

Kielhofner G 1980a A model of human occupation, part 2. Ontogenesis from the perspective of temporal adaptation. American Journal of Occupational Therapy 34(10): 657–663

Kielhofner G 1980b A model of human occupation, part 3. Benign and vicious cycles. American Journal of Occupational Therapy 34(11): 731–737

Kielhofner G (ed) 1985 A model of human occupations. Williams & Wilkins, Baltimore

Kielhofner G 1988 The model of human occupation workbook. Workshops, London, Edinburgh, York

Kielhofner G 1992 Conceptual foundations of occupational therapy. F A Davis, Philadelphia

Kielhofner G 1995 A model of human occupation theory and application, 2nd edn. Williams and Wilkins, Baltimore

Kielhofner G, Burke J P 1980 A model of human occupation, part 1. Conceptual framework and content. American Journal of Occupational Therapy 34(9): 572–581

Kielhofner G, Burke J P, Igi C H 1980 A model of human occupation, part 4. Assessment and intervention, American Journal of Occupational Therapy 34(12): 777–778

Kirshenbaum H, Henderson V L (eds) 1990 Carl Rogers dialogues. Constable, London

King L J 1974 A sensory integrative approach to schizophrenia. American Journal of Occupational Therapy 28: 529–536

Kings Fund Centre 1988 The problem orientated medical record (POMR): guidelines for therapists. Kings Fund Centre, London

Knowles M 1978 The adult learner: a neglected species. Gulf, Houston

Kortman B 1994 The eye of the beholder: models in occupational therapy. Australian Journal of Occupational Therapy 41: 115–122

Low M et al 1990 the Canadian occupational performance measure an outcome measure for occupational therapy, CJOT 52(2): 82–87

Low M et al 1992 Canadian occupational performance measure (Manual), 2nd edn. CAOT publications, Toronto

Levy L L 1993 Cognitive disability frame of reference. In: Willard and Sparkman's Occupational Therapy. Lippincott, Philadelphia

Lovell R B 1987 Adult learning. Croom Helm, London

Macdonald J 1990 The international course on conductive education at the Peto Andras State Institute for Conductive Education Budapest. British Journal of Occupational Therapy 53(7): 295–300

McColl M A, Pranger T 1994 Theory and practice in the occupational therapy guidelines for client centred practice CJOT 61(5): 250–259

McKay E A, Ryan S 1995 Clinical reasoning through storytelling: examining a student's case story on a fieldwork placement. British Journal of Occupational Therapy 58(6): 234–238

Maslow A H 1968 Towards a psychology of being. Van Nostrad, New York

Maslow A H 1970 Motivation and personality. Harper & Row, New York

Mattingly C, Fleming M H 1994 Clinical reasoning; forms of inquiry in a therapeutic practice. F A Davis, Philadelphia

McDonald E M 1964 Occupational Therapy in rehabilitation, 2nd edn. Bailliére Tindall, London

Miller R J, Walker K F 1993 Perspectives on theory for the practice of occupational therapy. Aspen, Gaithersburg

Mills D, Fraser C 1989 Therapeutic activities for the upper limb. Winslow Press, Bicester

Mocellin G 1988 A perspective on the principles and practice of occupational therapy. British Journal of Occupational Therapy

Mosey A C 1968 Recapitulation of ontogenesis: a theory for the practice of occupational therapy. American Journal of Occupational Therapy 22(5)

Mosey A C 1970 Three frames of reference for mental health. Slack, New Jersey

Mosey A C 1973 Activities therapy. Raven Press, New York

Mosey A C 1981 Occupational therapy: configuration of a profession. Raven Press, New York

Mosey A C 1986 Psychosocial components of occupational therapy. Raven Press, New York

Newell A 1977 On the analysis of human problem solving protocols. In: Johnson-Laird P N, Wason P C (eds) Thinking: readings in cognitive science. New Jersey

Norkin C C, White J 1985 Measurement of joint motion. F A Davis, Philadelphia

Pedretti L (ed) Occupational therapy: practice skills for physical dysfunction, 2nd edn. C V Mosby

Pedretti L W, Zolton B 1990 Occupational therapy: practice skills for physical dysfunction, 3rd edn. C V Mosby

Perry W G 1970 Forms of intellectual and ethical development in the college years: a scheme. Holt, Rinehart & Winston, New York

Priestly R et al 1978 Social skills and personal problem solving. Tavistock Publications, London

Reed K L 1984 Models of practice in occupational therapy. Williams & Wilkins, Baltimore

Reed K L, Sanderson S 1992 Concepts of occupational therapy, 3rd edn. Williams and Wilkins, Baltimore

Remocker A J, Storch E T 1982 Action speaks louder. Churchill Livingstone, Edinburgh

Robertson E 1984 The role of the occupational therapist in a psychotherapeutic setting. British Journal of Occupational Therapy 47(4)

Rogers C 1983 Freedom to learn for the 80s. Merrill, Columbus Ohio

Rogers C 1984 Client centred therapy: its current practice, implications and theory. Houghton Miffin, Boston

Rogers C 1986 On becoming a person. Constable

Rogers J C, Holm M B, 1991 Occupational therapy diagnostic reasoning: a component of clinical reasoning. American Journal of Occupational Therapy 45(11): 1045–1053

Ross M, Burdick D 1981 Sensory Integration. Slack, New Jersey

Slater D Y, Cohn E S 1991 Staff development through the analysis of practice. American Journal of Occupational Therapy 45(11): 1038–1044

Tornebohm H 1991 What is worth knowing in occupational therapy? American Journal of Occupational Therapy 45: 451–454

Trombley C A 1989 Occupational therapy for physical dysfunction, 3rd edn. Williams & Wilkins, Baltimore

Turner A (ed) 1987 The practice of occupational therapy, 2nd edn. Churchill Livingstone, Edinburgh

Turner A (ed) 1996 The principles, skills and practice of occupational therapy, 4th edn. Churchill Livingstone, Edinburgh

Turner A (ed) 1992 The principles, skills and practice of occupational therapy, 3rd edn. Churchill Livingstone, Edinburgh

Yallom I D 1975 Theory and practice of group psychotherapy. Basic Books, New York

Yallom I D 1983 In-patient group psychotherapy. Basic Books, New York

Young M 1984 Models of practice for occupational therapy. British Journal of Occupational Therapy 47(12): 381–382

Young M, Quinn 1992 Theories and practice of occupational therapy. Churchill Livingstone, Edinburgh

Yule W, Carr J Behaviour modification for the mentally handicapped. Croom Helm, London

Yura H, Walsh M S 1988 The nursing process, assessing, planning, implementing, evaluating, 5th edn. Appleton and Lange, Norwalk Conn

Watts N 1990 Handbook of clinical teaching. Churchill Livingstone, Edinburgh

Watts F, Bennett D (eds) 1981 Principles of psychiatric rehabilitation. Wiley, Chichester.

Weed L L 1968 Medical records that guide and teach. New England Journal of Medicine 278: 593–599

Weed L L 1969 Medical records, medical education and patient care. Western Reserve University, Cleveland

Wilcock A A 1986 Occupational therapy approaches to stroke. Churchill Livingstone, Edinburgh

Whittaker D S 1985 Using groups to help people. Routledge & Kegan, London

Willson M 1984 Occupational therapy in short-term psychiatry, 2nd edn. Churchill Livingstone, Edinburgh

Willson M 1987 Occupational therapy in long-term psychiatry, 2nd edn. Churchill Livingstone, Edinburgh

Wing J K, Morris B (eds) 1981 Handbook of psychiatric rehabilitation. Oxford University Press, Oxford

Zoltan B, Seive E, Freishtat B 1986 Perceptual and cognitive dysfunction in the adult stroke patient, 2nd edn. Slack

Glossary

Note

The Glossary includes words defined in the text, and words used in connection with models and professional practice. It does not include medical or psychological terms which may readily be found in specialist dictionaries, but a few terms which may be difficult to find, or are notoriously confusing, are defined. Where there are two meanings, or where several, differing definitions exist, the alternatives are given.

Sources for definitions

Proliferating definitions are of no use to the student, or to the profession. Where clear definitions exist which are compatible with the text, I have used these, and sources are indicated as shown in the code below. Those marked (RH) are my own.

(At)	Atkinson et al 1993 Introduction to psychology, 11th edn. Harcourt Brace Javanovich
(Cr)	Creek J (ed) 1990 Occupational therapy and mental health: principles, skills and practice. Churchill Livingstone, Edinburgh
(WS)	Hopkins H L, Smith H D (eds) 1988 Willard and Spackman's occupational therapy, 7th edn. Lippincott, Philadelphia
(Kh)	Kielhofner G 1992 Conceptual foundations of occupational therapy. F A Davis, Philadelphia
(Kh95)	Kielhofner G 1995 A model of human occupation theory and application. Williams and Wilkins, Baltimore
(Lov)	Lovell R B 1987 Adult Learning. Croom Helm, London
(Polgar)	Polgar S, Thomas S A 1991 Introduction to research in the health sciences, 2nd edn. Churchill Livingstone, Edinburgh
(R)	Reed K L, Sanderson S R 1992 Concepts of occupational therapy, 3rd edn. Williams and Wilkins, Baltimore
(COD)	Sykes J B (ed) 1982 The concise Oxford dictionary, 7th edn. Clarendon Press, Oxford
( )	*Other authors given in brackets.*

GENERAL GLOSSARY

Algorithm   A diagrammatic method of illustrating the stages and alternative decisions at each stage in a process. (RH)

Autonomy   Personal freedom; freedom of the will. (COD)
The ability to act or perform according to one's own volition or direction. (R)
Quality of being self-governing and self-determining. (WS)

Behaviour   Those activities of an organism that can be observed by another organism (or by instrumentation). Included within behaviour are verbal reports made about subjective, conscious experiences. (At)

Behaviourism   Study of human actions by analysis into stimulus and response. (COD)
A branch of psychology which attempts to discover the laws that describe behaviour by relying exclusively on observable data. (Lov)

Cognition   An individual's thoughts, knowledge, interpretations, understanding or ideas. (At)

Cognitive Processes   Mental processes of perception, memory and information processing by which the individual acquires information, makes plans and solves problems. (At)

Clinical reasoning   Cognitive processes involving information processing, problem solving, judgement and decision making, used by clinicians when identifying and interpreting features of the individual's situation in order to form a diagnosis of the problem and determine treatment goals and interventions. (RH)

Concept   A system of learned responses which enables us to organize and interpret data. (Lov)
Idea of a class of objects. (COD)
A general idea or meaning usually mediated by a work, symbol or sign. (R)

Countertransference   Conscious or unconscious responses of therapist to the patient determined by the therapist's need; transferred feelings, not necessarily relevant to the real situation. (WS)

Defence mechanism   Unconscious intrapsychic process, e.g. denial, introjection, projection, rationalization. (WS)

Determinism   Doctrine that human action is not free but determined by motives regarded as external forces acting on the will. (COD)

Development   The progressive and continuous change in

shape, function and integration of the body from birth to death. (R)

Disability Loss or impairment of one or more bodily organs with corresponding functional loss. (COD)
The reduction of functional ability to lead a fruitful daily life. It is the result not only of mental and/or physical impairment but also of the individual's adjustment to this. *Note*: This term must be considered along with impairment, handicap and incapacity. The various terms have not always been clearly distinguished from one another. In general English usage, disability and handicap are often used interchangeably, and there is a tendency to equate both terms with the more severe and obvious conditions. A logical sequence might be as follows:

Impairment The basic pathological condition. An impairment may be so minor as not to interfere materially with functional ability, or it may be possible to correct or restore function. If an impairment is major, and not capable of correction it will produce:

Disability The loss or reduction of functional ability. The effect of this will depend on the individual's personal circumstances and requirements: it may well amount to:

Handicap The disadvantage or restriction of activity caused by disability. (WHO)

Divergent thinking A cognitive operation in which the subject thinks in different directions. The quality of divergent thought is judged in terms of the quantity, variety and originality of the ideas produced. (Lov)

Dualism Theory recognizing two independent principles — mind and matter. (COD)

Dyadic interaction *Of skills*: Abilities in relationships to peers, subordinates and authority figures; demonstrating trust, respect and warmth; perceiving and responding to needs and feelings of others; engaging in and sustaining interdependent relationships; communicating feelings. (R)

Eclectic Borrowing freely from various sources. (COD)

Ecology (human) Study of interaction of persons with their environment. (COD)

Empirical Founded on practical experience but not proved scientifically; based on observable fact or objective experience. (WS)

Ethnography *In research*: A descriptive qualitative study, often of an individual or situation, usually written from the perspective of the participant(s) in the first person. (Polgar 1991)

Ethnomethodology A qualitative approach to research which involves the study of social processes associated with ways in which people perceive, describe and explain the world. (Polgar 1991)

Existentialism Philosophical theory emphasizing existence of the individual person as free and responsible agent determining his own development. (COD)

Experiential learning A view that all learning is best gained by direct experience, which must be meaningful to the learner. (RH)

Feedback Modification or control of a process or system by its results and effects especially by difference between desired and actual result. (COD)
Information about the consequences of the actions taken by a person performing a skill. (Lov)

Gestalt Perceived organized whole that is more than the sum of its parts. (COD)

Gestalt psychology A system of psychological theory concerned primarily with perception that emphasizes pattern, organization, wholes and field properties. (At)

Habilitation The encouragement and stimulation of the development and acquisition of skills and functions not previously attained. (R)

Handicap Having less than normal ability or having an anatomical or functional defect which makes it difficult for one to compete with one's peers. (R) (see also Disability)

Heuristic Quality that encourages further discovery or investigation. (WS)
In problem solving, a strategy that can be applied to a variety of problems that usually, but not always, provides a correct solution. (At)

Holistic *Of therapy*: A conscious attempt to view all aspects of a client's problem or situation as a gestalt, and to treat all aspects accordingly. (RH)
Relating to or stressing the functional relationships of parts and wholes. In health care holistic thinking considers the person's whole life circumstances and not just the disease or trauma. (Kh)

Humanism System which views man as a responsible and progressive intellectual being. (COD)
A system of beliefs and a theoretical approach that is concerned with what it means to become fully human. (Cr)

Humanistic medicine Medical practice and culture that respects and incorporates the concepts of humanism in which the consumer and professional share responsibility for maintaining or regaining health and well-being. (R)

Humanistic psychology A psychological approach that emphasizes the uniqueness of human beings: it is concerned with subjective experience and human values. (At)

Hypothesis Proposition made as a basis for reasoning without assumption of its truth; supposition made as a starting point for further investigation from known facts. (COD)

Illuminative study One which recounts subjective personal experience with a view to providing insights into causes, processes and the effectiveness of procedures. (RH)

Information processing *In cognitive psychology*: The mental processes required to store, retrieve and make use of information. Models which explain or describe this process. (RH)

Input Information entering a system from the environment. (RH)

Kinesiology The study of human movement. (RH)

Mechanistic *Relates to*: Doctrine that all natural phenomena, including life, allow mechanical explanation by physics and chemistry. (COD)
The tendency to see the mind or body as machine-like in their operations. (RH)
A theory which holds that to explain any phenomenon one must discover its parts, how they are put together and how they interact. (Kh95)

Modelling Setting an example for imitation (usually, of social behaviour). (RH)

Monism Any of the theories which deny the duality of matter and mind. (COD)

Naturalistic method Techniques of research conducted in normal environments without artificial controls. (RH)

Object relations The ability of the person to invest feelings and emotions in other persons or objects. (R)

Ontogenesis Origin and development of an individual. (COD)

Ontogeny Development of an individual over the passage of time. (RH)

Open systems theory Living organisms are dynamic, self-organizing entities, exhibiting ongoing interaction with their environments. (Kh95)

Organismic A view of reality which emphasizes the subjective, interactive and holistic nature of human experience. (see Holistic; Phenomenological) (RH)

Output The product of the processes of a system. (RH)
Action of the system which produces a change in the environment; mental, physical and social aspects of occupation. (Kh)

Perception Mental process by which intellectual, sensory and emotional data are organized meaningfully; the process of conscious recognition and interpretation of sensory stimuli. (WS)

Phenomenological Relating to the study of *phenomena* — things which are perceived and reported as part of individual conscious subjective experience. (RH)

Philosophy Seeking after wisdom or knowledge, especially that which deals with ultimate reality or the most general causes and principles of things and ideas and human perception and knowledge of them. (COD)
A critique and analysis of fundamental beliefs as they come to be conceptualized and formalized. (R)

Physiology Science of functions and phenomena of living organisms and their parts. (COD)

Problem oriented medical records (POMR) A system for recording problems affecting a patient and planning and organizing action to resolve these. (RH)

Problem solving A set of cognitive strategies used to resolve difficulties. (RH)

Profession An occupation characterized by a defined body of knowledge and expertise, whose practitioners espouse a code of ethics and responsible conduct in relation to their clients. (RH)

Proprioception Appreciation of position, balance and changes in equilibrium of a body part during movement as a result of stimulus to receptors within body tissue such as muscle, tendons and joints. (WS)

Psychoanalysis A therapeutic system for the treatment of mental disorder based on the principles of analytical psychology, aimed at investigating interaction of conscious and unconscious elements in the mind and bringing the latter into consciousness. (RH)

Psychotherapy Treatment of personality maladjustment or mental disorders by psychological means, usually, but not exclusively, through personal consultation. (At)

Psychology Science of the nature, functions and phenomena of the human mind. (COD)

Quantitative methods An approach to research that emphasizes the collection of numerical data and the statistical analysis of hypotheses proposed by the researcher. (Polgar)

Qualitative methods An approach to research that emphasizes the non-numerical and interpretive analysis of social phenomena. (Polgar)

Quality assurance Activities and programmes intended to insure the quality of care in a defined medical setting or programme. (R)

Rehabilitation Restoration to a disabled individual of maximum independence commensurate with his limitations by developing his residual capacities. (WS)
The combined and coordinated use of medical, social, educational and vocational measures for training or retraining the individual to the highest possible level of functional ability. (WHO)

Rehabilitative services Those activities and procedures designed to assist a physically or mentally disabled individual to achieve or maintain the highest attainable level of function through an evaluation and treatment programme providing, under physician direction, one or a combination of medical, paramedical, psychological, social and vocational services determined by the needs of the patient.

Reliability The extent to which a test or measurement is reproducable by different people or at different times. (RH)

Self-actualization The capacity of the individual to achieve a life which fulfils potentials and offers satisfaction and personal meaning. (RH)

SOAP Heading used in POMR; Subjective; Objective; Analysis; Plan. (RH)

Standardized test One that has known characteristics, especially known levels of reliability and validity. (Polgar)

Systems theory The basis for the study of the operation of systems. Systems may be described as 'hard', i.e. of a fixed, mechanical nature; or 'soft', i.e. changing, dynamic interactions between people and environments. The operation of a system is usually described in terms of input, output, throughput and feedback. (RH)

Taxonomy Principles of classification. (COD) (Especially used in botany, biology and education)

Teleological Purposeful; relating to the view that developments are due to the purpose or design that is served by them. (COD)

Temporal Of, in, or denoting time. (COD)

Theory A system of assumptions, accepted principles and rules of procedure devised to analyse, predict or otherwise explain the nature or behaviour of a specific set of phenomena. (R)
Set of logically interrelated statements used to explain observed events. A proposed explanation whose status is still conjectural in contrast to well established propositions that are regarded as reporting matters of fact. (WS)

Transference *In Psychoanalysis:* Projection of feelings, thoughts or wishes on to another who has come to represent someone from the past; inappropriate feelings applied in present context. (WS)

Validity The extent to which a test measures what it is intended to measure. (Polgar)

TERMS USED IN OCCUPATIONAL THERAPY

Activity A specific action, function or sphere of action that involves learning or doing by direct experience. (R)
An integrated sequence of tasks which takes place on a specific occasion, during a finite period, for a particular purpose. (RH)

Activity programme A programme designed to encourage individual and/or group participation through organized events for the purpose of maintaining or improving skills, roles or interactions. (RH)

Activity analysis Dissection of an activity into its component tasks and the evaluation of therapeutic potential and relevance to the treatment plan; investigating the objective or subjective performance components. (RH)

Activity synthesis Combining and adapting components of

an activity with components of the environment to assess performance, enhance skills or produce a desired therapeutic outcome. (RH)

Adaptation to activity Modification of features such as sequence, complexity, positioning, location, use of tools, construction of equipment, to meet treatment objectives, or to improve performance.

Adaptation 1. Any change in structure, form or habits of an organism to suit new environment. Those changes experienced by an individual which lead to adjustment (WS)
2. An alteration made by a therapist to an environment or an object in order to provide therapy or to improve the client's ability to function. (RH)

Adaptive behaviour The integration of skill areas with socially accepted values to accomplish occupations and tasks. (R)

Aim A brief statement of the general purpose which treatment or intervention will be planned to achieve. (RH)

Approach Ways and means of putting theory into practice. (RH)

Assessment The process of collecting information, including subjective and objective data which are relevant to the preparation of an intervention plan. (R)

Competence Skilled and adequately successful completion of a task or activity. (RH)

Core skills Basic components of professional practice which remain relatively constant although adapted by the use of frames of reference, models and approaches. (RH)

Diversional activities Those designed to alleviate boredom and to provide an enjoyable interest, without specific therapeutic intent. (RH)

Dysfunction A temporary or chronic inability to engage in the roles, relationships and occupations expected of a person of a comparable age, sex and culture. (RH)
Inability to maintain the self within the environment at a satisfactory standard because of lack of skills necessary for coping with the current situation. (Cr)

Environmental adaptation Changing the physical or social features of an environment to enhance performance, promote or restrict a behaviour, or provide therapy. (RH)

Environmental analysis Observation of features in the physical or social environment and interpretation of their significance or patient performance or therapy.

Environmental demand The combined effect of elements in the environment to produce expectations for certain human actions and reactions. (RH)

Facilitation 1. *Of groups*: Helpful, non-directive leadership style. (RH)
2. *Of neurodevelopmental techniques*: Specific treatment which promotes sensorimotor integration and the recovery or development of normal patterns of movement. (RH)

Frame of reference Belief system based on conceptual models; in therapy, organized basis of theory, delineation of function and dysfunction, evaluation and treatment approaches, postulates regarding change. (WS)
A set of interrelated, internally consistent concepts, definitions and postulates derived from or compatible with empirical data providing a systematic description or proscription for particular designs of the environment for the purpose of facilitating evaluation and effecting change. (Mosey)
A set of basic assumptions necessary to determine the subject matter to be studied and the orientation towards such study. (R)

A system of theories serving to orient and give particular meaning to a set of circumstances which provides a coherent conceptual basis for therapy. (Creek, Foster, Turner and Hagedorn)

Functional ability (function/functional) The skill to perform activities in a normal or accepted manner. (SR)
Having the ability to perform competently the roles, relationships and occupations required in the course of daily life. (RH)

Grading Measurable increasing or decreasing of activity, graded by length of time, size, degree of strength required or amount of energy expended. (R)

Habituation subsystem An internal organization of information that disposes the system to exhibit recurrent patterns of behaviour. (Kh95)

Interpersonal *Of skills*: Those which are used for interactions between people. The level, quality and/or degree of dyadic and group interaction skills. (WS)

Intervention Action by the therapist on behalf of the client/patient. The process of putting the plan into action and carrying it out. (WS)

Intrapersonal *Of skills*: Those which operate within the mind and emotions of the individual. (RH)
The level, quality and/or degree of self-identity, self-concept and coping skills. (WS)

Meaningfulness *Of activities*: The individual's predisposition to find importance, security, sense of worth and purpose in certain forms of occupations. (Kh)

Medium (*pl. Media*) An agency or activity through which something is accomplished. An intervening substance through which something is transmitted or carried on. In OT, an activity or task having therapeutic potential. (R)

Mind/brain/body performance subsystem The organization of physical and mental constituents which together make up the capacity of occupational performance. (Kh95)

Modality A therapeutic agent/activity; the application of a therapeutic agent. (R) (syn. Medium)

Model A set of ideas derived from various fields of study which are organized to form a synthesis and integration of elements of theory and practice. (RH)
A representational tool which orders, categorizes and simplifies complex phenomena; describes the organization among parts. (Kh)
A simplified representation of the structure and content of a phenomenon or system that describes or explains the complex relationships between concepts within the system. (Cr)

Occupation a form of human endeavour which provides longitudinal organization or time and effort in a person's life. (RH)
Activity or task which engages a person's resources of time and energy. Specifically; self-maintenence, productivity and leisure. (R)
The human being's interaction with the environment which arises out of an innate urge towards exploration and mastery and the consequent ability to symbolize: the essence of human existence and adaptation. (Kh)
Any goal directed activity that has meaning for the individual and is composed of skills and values. (Cr)

Occupational behaviour Organization and action based on skills, knowledge and attitude to make functioning possible in life roles. (Reilly)

Occupational therapy The treatment of physical and psychiatric conditions through specific selected activities in order to help people to reach their maximum level of function in all aspects of daily life. (WFOT)

The restoration or maintenance of optimal functional independence and life satisfaction through the analysis and use of selected occupations that enable the individual to develop the adaptive skills required to support his life roles. (Cr)

The use of purposeful activity with individuals who are limited by physical illness or injury, psychosocial dysfunction, developmental or learning disabilities, poverty and cultural differences, or the ageing process in order to maximize independence, prevent disability and maintain health. AOTA

The prescription of occupations, interactions and environmental adaptations to enable the individual to regain, develop or retain the occupational skills and roles required to maintain personal well-being and to achieve meaningful personal goals and relationships appropriate to the relevant social and cultural setting. (RH)

Occupational performance Human behaviour having three areas: self-care, productivity and leisure which are based on the interaction of the individual's mental, physical, sociocultural and spiritual performance components. Model based on this concept. (adapted from Canadian Association of OT 1991)

Objective A precise statement of the purpose, process and outcome of therapy. (RH)

Paradigm Accepted examples of scientific practice which include law, theory appreciation and instrumentation and which represent a radically new conceptualization of the phenomena. (Kuhn)

A consensus of the most fundamental beliefs or assumptions of a field. The occupational therapy paradigm is the field's means of defining human beings and their problems in a way which suggests and provides a rationale for course of action to solve them. (Kh)

An agreed body of theory, explaining and rationalizing professional unity and practice, that incorporates all the profession's concerns, concepts and expertise and guides values and commitments. (Cr)

Performance skills Skills required for successful performance of the roles that are assumed by individuals in their lives. (WS)

Personal causation Self-perception of effectiveness within the environment. (Kh)

The individual's capacity to initiate action with the intent to affect the environment. (Cr)

Role A social or occupational identity which directs the individual's social, cultural and occupational behaviour and relationships.

Individuals typically require the capacity to carry out a variety of roles at any point in life. (RH)

Skill A specific ability or integrated set of abilities (e.g. motor, sensory, cognitive or perceptual) learnt and practised to a standard required for the effective performance of a task or subtask. (RH)

Skill analysis Analysis of a skill to identify the components required for its performance.

Subskill A primary component of a skill. (RH) (syn. Skill component)

Subtask A non-reducible component of a task. (RH) (syn. Task segment)

Task A stage in or component of an activity. (RH)

Techniques The body of specialized procedures and methods used in treatment. (RH)

Volition subsystem System of dispositions and self-knowledge that predisposes and enables person to anticipate, choose, experience and interpret occupational behaviour. (Kh95)

OCCUPATIONAL THERAPY TECHNIQUES

The definitions given below provide an explanation of some of the terms used in the text which may be unfamiliar to you. These definitions are my own, unless otherwise stated. This is not intended as a comprehensive list, but as an indication of some commonly used techniques, (although some are restricted to a speciality, e.g. paediatrics, learning disabilities, or to a specific frame of reference/approach).

Techniques may be practiced at different levels depending on the experience and degree of specialization of the therapist. A newly qualified therapist may have an understanding of the basic principles, and competence in frequently used techniques, but at a more advanced level the practitioner will normally require additional experience and training to become proficient and may need to work under close supervision until proficiency is attained.

Activities of daily living (ADL) assessment and training A period of objective appraisal of an individual's functional ability when performing necessary ADL, followed by a period of training or re-education in order to improve function.

Anxiety management Techniques having a cognitive and/or behavioural basis, used to help clients to monitor and control personal anxiety levels.

Assertion training Techniques which enable the individual to appreciate personal individuality and worth, to recognize personal feelings and needs and to express these in a socially acceptable manner. Training often employs group techniques and role-play.

Behaviour modification A method of psychotherapy based on learning principles, it uses techniques such as counter-conditioning, reinforcement and shaping to modify behaviour. (At) The objective is either to remove an unproductive, injurious or antisocial behaviour, or to promoting positive behaviour.

Behavioural rehearsal A cognitive technique in which the client acts out and practises behaviours which are found to be difficult or stressful before attempting them in reality, and develops solutions to problems.

Biofeedback Technique in which patient is made aware of unconscious or involuntary physiological processes and learns to control them. (WS)

Chaining Technique of teaching behaviour patterns by giving reinforcement for individual components of a behaviour which may be learnt separately and then linked to form a whole. *Backward chaining* is a form of errorless learning in which a task or behaviour is taught by commencing at the point of completion and working backwards to the start.

Cognitive behaviour therapy A psychotherapy approach that emphasizes the influence of a person's beliefs, thoughts and self-statements on behaviour. Combines behaviour therapy methods with those designed to change the way the individual thinks about self and events. (At)

Compensatory techniques Those used to compensate for a physical or cognitive deficit in performance: e.g. provision of adaptive equipment or environment, or teaching new methods of performing tasks.

Counselling The use of client centred techniques to enable the client to identify problems, feelings or conflicts and to reach solutions or decisions.

Desensitization Use of progressive exposure of the patient in a safe environment to a stimulus which provokes acute anxiety or other negative reaction until the point is reached where the patient can tolerate the stimulus without becoming dysfunctional.

Energy conservation Techniques including time management, time and motion study, problem solving and environmental planning enabling a patient to make maximum functional use of limited potential for energy expenditure.

Errorless learning Teaching techniques (cognitive/behavioural) which teach concepts or skills by presenting material or instruction in such a way that the possibility of failure by the learner is eliminated.

Functional assessment May include ADL assessment (see above) or may refer to specific observation and/or measurement of aspects of physical function (e.g. grip strength, mobility, range of movement).

Gaming The use of scenarios, tasks, or problem solving exercises to provide groups of people with personal experience of group processes, deicision making mechanisms, leadership styles, or the effects of emotions, attitudes and preconceptions.

Gentle teaching A humanistic method of teaching people with learning disabilities whilst maintaining their human rights and enabling them to have an accepted place in society.

Guided fantasy Techniques in which a group leader, by means of words, images or music, provides stimulus for each individual to construct mental images, stories or journeys leading to insightful exploration of personal symbols, fantasies, desires, emotions or choices.

Home adaptations The design and provision of physical alterations to an individual's home in order to promote independent living.

Homework A term used in some cognitive techniques where a patient is given tasks to do at home usually involving a record of results and personal reactions during and after the process.

Interviewing Techniques include formal, informal, structured and unstructured methods; interviews may be used to obtain information or to negotiate aims and objectives or to evaluate courses of action.

Industrial therapy Use of industrial work processes, frequently packing, assembly work, or clerical work, in a simulation of a realistic work environment, with nominal pay, to assess, promote or retrain work skills.

Joint protection Instructing patients in ways of managing personal, domestic or work activities in a manner which reduces or eliminates potentially damaging stresses on vulnerable joints. Particularly used in the management of arthritic conditions.

Lifestyle planning Techniques which enable an individual to attain a balance between the occupational elements in his/her life (work, leisure, self-care, rest) in order to reduce stress, improve quality of life, develop potentials and attain relevant personal goals.

Milieu therapy A psychotherapeutic term meaning the modification of a physical and social environment such as that provided by a therapeutic community for treatment purposes.

Mobility training Instruction of a patient in the use of mobility equipment and wheelchairs.

Neurodevelopmental techniques Techniques used in the treatment of sensorimotor disorders which are based on the use of techniques such as reflex inhibition, positioning, and sensory stimulation (e.g. Bobath, Rood, PNF). (RH)

Orthotics Assessment for, design of and production and fitting of orthoses (splints) for functional or supportive purposes, often for the upper limb.

Pacing Techniques which enable the individual to perform activities or tasks in a preplanned manner, sticking to measurable personal targets, involving use of task analysis, timed activity, rest periods, alternating types of movement, in order to maximize effective performance and minimize undesirable consequences such as pain, stress on joints, or fatigue.

Perceptual training Techniques designed to train or re-educate perceptual functions such as discriminations of size, form, colour, laterality, by repeated practice.

Portage A developmentally based programme constructed by a therapist enabling a parent of a handicapped child to work with the child at home, using play and care activities to achieve defined goals.

Prosthetic training Techniques of instructing patients in the use of upper and lower limb prostheses following amputation.

Projective techniques The use of creative media, especially art, music, modelling, writing, in a manner which encourages personal interpretations of the material and facilitates exploration of personal experiences, symbols and feelings.

Psychodrama The use of dramatic techniques, e.g. role-play, improvization, mime, to construct or reconstruct scenarios of significance to the participants, or to engage them in experiences which will enable them to explore life themes, emotions, thoughts, reactions, relationships or defensive and coping mechanisms.

Reality orientation Used with dementing or brain damaged individuals to cue them into awareness of current time, place, persons and current circumstances. Can involve '24 hour' and 'classroom' techniques.

Relaxation Various methods involving techniques of voluntary physical or mental control designed to produce physical and mental relaxation and relieve the effects of stress or anxiety.

Reminiscence therapy (nostalgia therapy) Techniques used with dementing individuals or very elderly people in which objects from the past—photos, music, clothes, objects—are used as triggers for discussion and reflection and the sharing or validation of personal experiences and memories.

Retirement planning Techniques which enable people who have/are about to retire from work to develop a balanced and fulfilling repertoire of occupations and interests, and to maintain a healthy lifestyle.

Role-play Use of dramatic techniques and improvization to enable patients to act out roles or situations which they wish to explore, either to gain insight into difficulties or to improve coping skills.

Room management techniques A means of providing individual attention to members of a large group for short periods, making best use of available staff and their skills, and the possibly limited attention span of participants. Typically one person acts as 'room manager' coordinating therapy, whilst another looks after physical care needs, or disturbances, and one or more others spend a few minutes with each group member in turn, working for a predetermined objective.

Sensory re-education Usually carried out to restore sensitivity and discrimination of touch in the hand following peripheral nerve injury; the patient is trained to recognize a variety of progressively finer and more similar textures by touch alone.

Social modelling Shaping behaviour or attitudes by enabling the learner to observe others performing competently and gaining suitable rewards or approval for such performance.

Social skills training Educational programmes designed to improve skills of interaction and acceptable social behaviour. May use social modelling, role-play and behavioural rehearsal.

Stress management A variety of cognitive and behavioural techniques used to enable the individual to recognize signs of personal stress and to adopt positive preventative and coping strategies to reduce this.

Token economy A form of behavioural modification in which the patient is rewarded for fulfilling a specified behavioural contract by 'tokens' which are usually tradeable for goods or privileges (a behavioural technique which is now seldom used).

Vocational (work) assessment Objective appraisal of a person's abilities to perform a previous (or future) job, which may include evaluation of the need for training or the provision of compensatory equipment or environmental adaptations.

Appendix

The following list indicates some of the general areas of assessment, and the types of techniques used within each of the approaches described.

Table of assessment techniques used within models and approaches

Approach	Assessment General Areas (e.g.s)	Techniques
Activities of daily living	Personal ADL Domestic ADL Need for aids	Observation; use of checklists and inventories; self-rating questionnaires; interview
Graded activities approach	Range of movement Strength of movement Speed of movement Dexterity/coordination Stamina Sensation Hand function — prehension Functional limitation Need for orthosis Use of prosthesis	Observation and physical examination; use of physical measurement equipment; checklists and record charts; unstructured or structured interview
Compensatory approach	Need for adaptive equipment or alterations to social or physical environment	Observation and testing measurement
Behavioural modification	Performance skills, e.g. personal care skills; communication skills; social skills; physical skills Abnormal responses, e.g. challenging behaviour; self mutilation; aggression	A variety of standardized validated tests of performance and behaviour. Several such tests are marketed, but some are only available for use by OTs with special training. Informal tests with a behavioural format may be used. Structured interview.
Cognitive perceptual	Apraxia Perception of objects, time, place, person Temporal orientation Agnosia Problem solving Organization Attitudes and values Flexibility/rigidity Memory Attention/concentration Intellectual abilities—numeracy, literacy	There are many validated cognitive tests but OT may need special training to use some of these. Unstandardized tests often used for perceptual deficits Several OT tests available (e.g. Rivermead, COTNAB). Full cognitive assessment is best done by a clinical psychologist. Structured interview, Performance tests

Approach	Assessment General Areas (e.g.s)	Techniques
Cognitive behavioural	Self-perceptions Links between behaviour and thoughts/feelings Level of anxiety/depression	Locus of control Self-efficacy Perceptions of past/future Psychological tests measuring anxiety, depression, stress etc. Level of engagement in activities
Analytical	Connections between unconscious feelings etc. and reality Perception of self Perception of others Object relations Use of symbols	Projective tests Personality tests Standardized assessments are not generally used by OTs in this approach. Some tests use projective, associative and symbolic media. Personality tests can only be used by OTs with special training. Unstructured interview.
Group work	Perception of self Perception of others Communication skills Assertion skills Level of stress Level of anxiety Social skills Reactions and interactions in groups	Some standardized tests are available for skills assessment; otherwise observation of the patient in interactive settings is used. Unstructured interview.
Client centred *Student centred*	Assessment by a person external to the client/student is largely irrelevant within this model, but self-assessment tests may be used to help to define problem areas, formulate future goals or measure progress. Interviews use client centred, reflective techniques.	

Processes of change

Rehabilitation	Rehabilitative assessments are functionally based and aimed at identifying deficits and charting recovery. Assessments tend to be related to either the chosen approach or technique, or to a specific occupational area—see elsewhere on this list. Structured or unstructured interviews often used.	
Development	Chronological v. actual developmental levels in performance skills—motor, sensory, perceptual, cognitive, interactive.	Tests are frequently standardized and many formal tests are sold for use in paediatrics. Structured or unstructured interviews.
Education	Assessment of educational attainment, except at a very basic level is not within the remit of an OT and should be referred to an educationist or educational psychologist. Tests used by OTs in this context tend to be cognitive, behavioural or occupational (see elsewhere on this list).	
Adaptation	Specific tests for 'adaptability' have not been designed, but those listed under cognitive-behavioural may be appropriate, together with tests measure rigidity/flexiblity and attitudes to change.	
Problem based process model	Depends on the approach chosen—see above.	

OT models

Adaptive skills	Assessment of developmental level in six performance areas: Sensory integration Cognition Perception Dyadic interaction Group interaction Self identity	Standardized tests devised for use within the model interviews

Approach	Assessment General Areas (e.g.s)	Techniques
Adaptation through occupations	Evaluation of physical; psychosocial; developmental and environmental problems. Skill development Chained behaviour Information skills Problem solving skills	Observation of performance; interview; informal testing; testing of specific skills; standardized tests as appropriate simulated tasks; measurement; timing.
Human occupations	Measurements of skills as defined by the model. Participation in occupations (past, present, future) Self-perceptions related to occupations	Observation and performance tests; a number of tests have been developed: Assessment of Motor and Process Skills (AMPS) Assessment of Communication and Interactive Skills (ACIS) Volitional questionnaire Self-report checklists and questionnaires: roles; interests; occupational questionnaire NIH Activity Record Self-assessment of occupational functioning (SADF) Interviews and detailed history taking are important, some with standardized formats, e.g. occupational case analysis interview and rating scale; assessment of occupational functioning; occupational performance history interview
Canadian occupational performance model	Assessment of performance components: physical, mental, sociocultural, spiritual.	The Canadian Occupational Performance Measure (COPM)
	Assessment of task functioning	Other observational or performance tests as required by the problem/approach
	Assessment of occupational performance; self-care; productivity leisure	
Cognitive disabilities	Assessment of cognitive level within terms of model	Allen cognitive level test Lower cognitive level test Object classification test Routine task history interview (structured interview and patient tasks) Also uses observation of functional/social performance.
Activities health	Detailed history of past, present and intended participation in activities.	Structured interview and observations Self-rated assessments Idiosyncratic activities configuration (includes analysed activities schedule)
	Assessments of skills and functional abilities	Usual methods

Occupational areas

Some OT assessments are related to occupational areas rather than to a model, although probably used within the context of one.

Activities of daily living (see ADL approach)

Work	Skills, knowledge, attitudes and habits required for work. Specific eg: Work tolerance	Observation Performance tests Checklists and rating scales Some standardized tests

Approach	Assessment General Areas (e.g.s)	Techniques
	Time keeping Work related skills — motor; cognitive; sensory; interpersonal Numeracy; literacy Assessment of work place environment Work aptitudes	Structured and unstructured interviews Full work aptitude assessment is best referred to an occupational psychologist or for vocational guidance
Leisure	Skills, interests and attitudes related to leisure, Attitudes/values Use of time/ability to plan Interests inventory Self-perception Mapping of leisure participation	Questionnaires and checklists, often self-rating Structured and unstructured interviews

Q Useful exercises in connection with this section:

1 List the assessment procedures which you are currently using. Does the list indicate a preferred model?
2 Do you use/have you seen in use any standardized or validated tests?
3 Obtain a selection of OT assessment forms and procedures and take a critical look at these. How clear are they? Do they look professionally presented? How valid do you think the results of the assessment can be considered to be?
4 If you think that a form or procedure could be improved how would you do this? Try making up a new version.

Index

References in italic are to the glossary section. Abbreviations: AFR – applied frames of reference; OT – occupational therapy

V